LOW-FODMAP DIET COOKBOOK

2100 DAYS OF EASY & TASTY RECIPES FOR DIGESTIVE DISORDER RELIEF AND IBS MANAGEMENT | INCLUDES A 60-DAY MEAL PLAN FOR OPTIMAL WELL-BEING + 4 BONUSES

JENNIFER NALLEY

Scan the QR code to access your 3 digital bonuses.

🔥 Bonus 1: 60 Day Meal Plan

🔥 Bonus 2: Emotional Well-being Tips

🔥 Bonus 3: Low Fodmap grocery shopping list

TABLE OF CONTENTS

INTRODUCTION

Welcome to Your Path to Digestive Health

Embarking on a journey towards better digestive health can often feel like navigating a treacherous path where every turn brings a new challenge. This is a voyage I know all too well. For years, I struggled with unsettling and painful symptoms that made daily activities cumbersome and sometimes unbearable. The discomfort of bloating, the unpredictability of IBS, and the constant pain were my everyday companions, making me dread meals that most people would enjoy without a second thought. It was during these trying times that I stumbled upon a beacon of hope—the LOW-FODMAP diet.

My introduction to the LOW-FODMAP diet was not unlike many others—born out of necessity and a desperate search for relief. Like many, my journey began in the doctor's office with a list of symptoms and a growing sense of frustration. The usual advice on eating healthily seemed ineffective, and the myriad of tests only pointed to 'IBS,' a label as broad as it was unhelpful. It was only when a friend, who had faced similar gastrointestinal battles shared her success with the LOW-FODMAP diet that I felt a flicker of hope.

The LOW-FODMAP diet, which stands for Fermentable Oligo-, Di-, Mono-saccharides, And Polyols, targets foods that are difficult to digest. These are not obscure, rarely consumed ingredients but are present in many common foods, from garlic and onions to wheat and apples. The diet involves a meticulous process of eliminating these foods temporarily and then systematically reintroducing them to identify personal triggers. It's a tailored approach, recognizing that digestive health is deeply personal and that what harms one may not harm another.

Starting the diet was daunting. The thought of overhauling my eating habits was overwhelming, especially when faced with the long list of restrictions. However, the potential reward of symptom relief kept me motivated. I began by eliminating all high-FODMAP foods, a stage known as the elimination phase. Those first few weeks were a revelation. Gradually, the daily discomfort began to fade, replaced by a sense of normalcy I had almost forgotten was possible.

As I progressed to the reintroduction phase, the diet's true value became apparent. I learned how my body reacted to different foods and discovered specific triggers that I could avoid or limit. This wasn't just about cutting out foods; it was about learning to understand and manage my digestive health actively.

The benefits of the LOW-FODMAP diet extend beyond physical relief. Emotionally, the feeling of control over my body and health was empowering. After years of helplessness, being proactive in managing my symptoms brought a profound sense of relief. Each meal became a choice, an opportunity to either nourish myself or to slip back into discomfort. The power of that choice was transformative.

However, the LOW-FODMAP diet is not a panacea, nor is it a life sentence of strict food avoidance. It's a tool—one of many in the quest for better health. For me, it was a critical step that allowed me to redefine my relationship with food. It taught me that dietary changes could lead to real, tangible improvements in quality of life. The journey through the phases of the LOW-FODMAP diet was interspersed with challenges and learning curves, but each step brought more understanding and greater control.

The community around the LOW-FODMAP diet also proved invaluable. Connecting with others who were navigating the same complex dietary changes offered support and reassurance that I wasn't alone in this journey. Through community forums, social media groups, and discussions, I found recipes, advice, and the kind of understanding that only those who've faced similar struggles can offer.

Today, as I share this path with you, my hope is that you, too, can experience the profound relief and empowerment that the LOW-FODMAP diet can offer. Whether you are at the beginning of your journey, struggling with symptoms without a clear cause, or you are an experienced dietary navigator looking for new solutions, the LOW-FODMAP diet offers a structured, evidence-based approach to improving digestive health.

Why This Cookbook? The Journey to Physical and Emotional Well-being

This cookbook is born out of a profound understanding that managing digestive health is as much about nurturing the body as it is about healing the mind. For countless individuals grappling with IBS and other digestive disorders, the daily reality includes not only physical discomfort but also significant emotional distress. The interplay between the gut and your emotional health is substantial, with each influencing the other in a continuous loop. By addressing both, this cookbook aims to offer a holistic approach to managing digestive health, providing not just recipes but a pathway to a better quality of life.

The journey to creating this cookbook began with a simple realization: food should be a source of pleasure, not anxiety. Those of us who suffer from digestive disorders often face each meal with trepidation, wondering how much we will have to pay for indulging our appetites. This constant anxiety can lead to a fraught relationship with food, where eating becomes a source of stress rather than comfort. The recipes in this book are carefully designed to eliminate common triggers of digestive discomfort, allowing you to enjoy delicious, nourishing meals without fear.

But this cookbook goes beyond providing safe recipes. It's crafted to reintroduce joy and relaxation into eating, transforming mealtime back into a soothing, restorative experience. Each recipe is more than a set of ingredients and instructions; it's a promise of enjoyment without discomfort, crafted with an understanding of both the physical requirements and emotional needs of those with sensitive digestive systems.

In crafting these recipes, great care was taken to ensure they were easy and quick to prepare. This consideration addresses another significant aspect of digestive disorders—the fatigue and lack of energy that often accompany symptoms. When a flare-up occurs, spending hours in the kitchen is the last thing anyone wants to do. This cookbook offers solutions that are practical and accessible, even on your worst days.

Moreover, the emotional support provided by this cookbook comes from its reassuring voice and empathetic understanding. It acknowledges the struggles faced by those with digestive issues and offers encouragement and hope. Each recipe is a small affirmation that you can take control of your health and enjoy life without compromise. It reinforces the message that your condition does not define you and that you can thrive despite it.

Additionally, the cookbook serves as a guide through the emotional landscape of dietary management. It provides tips on how to handle social eating, which is often a significant stressor for those on strict diets. Learning how to navigate restaurants, parties, and holiday meals without feeling isolated or deprived is crucial for emotional well-being. This book offers strategies for these situations, ensuring that readers feel equipped and confident in maintaining their dietary needs without missing out on life's celebratory moments.

The emotional relief that comes from following a diet that actually alleviates symptoms cannot be overstated. When you start to see real changes—less pain, more energy, fewer symptoms—the psychological boost is immense. This cookbook is designed to deliver those changes by guiding you through the LOW-FODMAP diet in a way that is clear, simple, and sustainable.

Moreover, this book emphasizes the importance of emotional well-being by including sections on how to deal with the mental and emotional aspects of living with a chronic digestive condition. It incorporates mindfulness practices, stress-reduction techniques, and advice on maintaining a positive outlook. These tools are invaluable since they assist in treating both the psychological effects and the physical symptoms of digestive issues.

How to Use This Book: A Guide to Navigating Your New Diet and Lifestyle

When you first open this cookbook, you might feel overwhelmed by the prospect of changing your diet and lifestyle. But fear not. This book is designed as a friendly guide to help you smoothly transition into a LOW-FODMAP lifestyle, a proven approach to managing digestive discomfort associated with IBS and other related conditions. Here's how you can best utilize the content of this book to ensure you achieve optimal results and truly transform your relationship with food.

Begin by reading the introductory chapters thoroughly. These sections are crucial as they lay the groundwork for understanding the why and how of the LOW-FODMAP diet. They provide essential background information that will help you grasp the scientific basis of the diet, the types of foods involved, and the reasons behind the recommended dietary changes. With this information, you will be able to make wise decisions moving forward and understand why some meals should be avoided and others should be enjoyed.

After familiarizing yourself with the basics, dive into the meal plans provided. These plans are carefully crafted to ease you into the diet without overwhelming you. Start with the 60-day meal plan, which is structured to introduce you to a variety of dishes while ensuring you adhere to the LOW-FODMAP guidelines. Take the uncertainty out of what to eat and when with daily meal plans that include breakfast, lunch, supper, and snacks. This plan is a tool to help you create consistent dietary habits that support digestive health, not merely a schedule.

As you follow the meal plan, begin experimenting with the recipes. Each recipe in this book is designed to be simple, with straightforward instructions and common ingredients that are easy to find in most supermarkets. Start with recipes that use ingredients you're already familiar with, gradually incorporating more novel ingredients as you become more comfortable with the diet. The recipes are not just meant to be followed but also understood;

as you cook, pay attention to how the ingredients complement each other to support your digestive health.

Use the bonus content to enhance your understanding and application of the LOW-FODMAP diet. This includes sections on how to reintroduce foods into your diet after the initial elimination phase, which is crucial for identifying your personal triggers. Follow the guidelines provided to introduce one food at a time, monitor your body's reactions, and adjust your diet accordingly. This personalized approach ensures that the diet works optimally for your unique digestive system.

The book also includes practical advice on how to incorporate the LOW-FODMAP diet into your everyday life. From tips on eating out and managing social situations to understanding how to read food labels, these insights will help you maintain your dietary changes in the long term without feeling restricted or isolated.

Moreover, take full advantage of the emotional support resources included in the book. Managing a chronic digestive condition can be emotionally taxing, and this book recognizes that. Sections dedicated to emotional well-being and stress management offer strategies to help you cope with the psychological aspects of living with digestive disorders. These resources are vital as they provide support that goes beyond dietary advice, addressing the holistic needs of individuals struggling with chronic conditions.

As you progress through the book, keep a journal of your experiences. Record what you eat, how you feel afterward, and any symptoms you notice. This record can be incredibly valuable for identifying which foods work best for you and which do not. It also serves as a motivational tool, allowing you to track your progress and see firsthand how your symptoms improve over time.

Understanding Digestive Disorders and IBS

IBS Management: Common Challenges and Solutions

Irritable Bowel Syndrome (IBS) presents a complex array of challenges that can transform simple daily activities into daunting tasks. Those who suffer from IBS often navigate a landscape filled with physical discomfort, emotional stress, and social obstacles. The variability of the condition means that each person's experience can differ significantly, making a one-size-fits-all solution impractical. However, understanding the common hurdles can pave the way for effective strategies to manage the condition.

One of the most immediate challenges of IBS is the physical discomfort and pain it causes. Abdominal cramps, bloating, gas, diarrhea, and constipation are frequent symptoms that can severely impact quality of life. Dietary adjustments are often necessary to manage these symptoms. The implementation of a LOW-FODMAP diet, which restricts foods like onions, garlic, certain fruits, and lactose, has been shown to significantly reduce symptoms for many sufferers. This diet minimizes the intake of fermentable oligosaccharides, disaccharides, monosaccharides, and polyols, which are carbohydrates that draw water into the intestinal tract and may cause fermentation and gas.

It can be difficult to follow such a rigorous diet, though, particularly when dining out or preparing food for a family that is not on the same diet. To tackle this, preparation is key. Planning meals ahead of time, carrying suitable snacks, and learning to spot hidden FODMAPs in restaurant menus and processed foods can help maintain this dietary approach without feeling isolated or deprived.

Another significant challenge is the unpredictability of flare-ups, which can lead to anxiety and stress about being far from familiar and safe restroom facilities. This anxiety can, in turn, exacerbate symptoms, creating a vicious cycle. To manage this, many people with IBS benefit from cognitive-behavioral strategies that help modify the thought patterns contributing to their stress. Techniques such as mindfulness meditation, deep breathing exercises, and yoga can also help alleviate both the psychological stress and the physical symptoms of IBS.

The social implications of IBS are not to be underestimated. The fear of a sudden need to use the restroom can deter sufferers from social outings and travel, leading to isolation and depression. Open communication with friends and family about one’s condition can foster understanding and support. Additionally, finding a support group, whether online or in person, can connect individuals with others facing similar challenges, providing a network of empathy and advice.

Workplace accommodations can also be a concern. It's beneficial for those with IBS to discuss their condition with their employer to find practical solutions that might include access to a private restroom or the flexibility to work from home during flare-ups. Legal protections, such as those provided under the Americans with Disabilities Act, may offer some support in managing these discussions and securing reasonable accommodations.

Fatigue often accompanies IBS, further complicating daily life. This can be managed through dietary adjustments to ensure proper nutrition despite restrictions. Supplements, such as vitamin D or magnesium, may be beneficial, but it's important to discuss these with a healthcare provider to ensure they are appropriate and safe. Regular, gentle exercise can also boost energy levels and improve overall digestive health.

Furthermore, the unpredictability of symptoms can complicate the management of IBS. Keeping a detailed food and symptom diary can help identify personal triggers and patterns, which, in turn, can predict potential flare-ups. This proactive approach allows individuals to adjust their plans and manage their activities around their condition more effectively.

Education about the condition is also crucial. Understanding that triggers and symptoms can vary widely among those with IBS can prevent discouragement and help sufferers continue to find the best personal management strategies. Staying informed about new research and treatments can also provide hope and additional options for managing the condition.

Lastly, the emotional toll of living with a chronic digestive disorder can be significant. Professional help from psychologists or counselors trained in chronic illness can help individuals develop coping strategies to deal with the frustrations and limitations that IBS can impose. This mental health support is crucial in maintaining emotional resilience and overall well-being.

While there are many obstacles associated with IBS, alleviation and an enhanced quality of life can be achieved through the creation of a thorough treatment plan that takes into account the mental and physical components of the illness. With the right strategies, support, and adjustments, those with IBS can lead active, fulfilling lives despite their condition.

The Role of Diet in Digestive Health

The significance of diet in managing digestive health cannot be overstated. What we eat directly impacts our digestive system, influencing everything from the balance of bacteria in our gut to the integrity of the gastrointestinal tract. The connection between food intake and digestive symptoms is well-documented in scientific research, highlighting the profound influence diet has on maintaining digestive health and managing disorders.

Every bite of food we take is a complex interaction of nutrients that affects our body. Foods are comprised of proteins, fats, carbohydrates, vitamins, and minerals that interact with our digestive system. Carbohydrates, for example, can be simple or complex, with the latter generally recommended for better digestive health because they are digested at a slower rate, leading to more stable blood sugar levels and a prolonged sense of fullness. Conversely, simple carbohydrates can cause rapid spikes in blood sugar and insulin levels, which can disrupt digestive processes and lead to discomfort.

Additionally, dietary fibers are essential for maintaining digestive health. To assist in making feces easier to move through the intestines, soluble fiber dissolves in water to create a gel-like material. Contrarily, insoluble fiber gives the stool more volume and facilitates food passage through the stomach and intestines more rapidly, which lowers the risk of constipation. In addition to being essential for preserving the integrity of the digestive tract, both forms of fiber support the gut microbiome, the population of bacteria that is essential for immune system regulation and food digestion.

One great illustration of how eating directly affects digestive health is the gut microbiota. This intricate web of fungi, bacteria, and viruses is necessary for breaking down food and obtaining nutrients. A diet full of a variety of nutrient-dense foods promotes a healthy microbiome, which benefits general health. In contrast, a diet heavy in processed foods and low in fiber can result in a less varied microbiome, which has been connected to a number of chronic illnesses, including type 2 diabetes and obesity, as well as digestive issues.

The scientific community has also explored the link between specific diets and digestive health. For instance, the LOW-FODMAP diet, which limits foods that are high in certain carbohydrates that draw water into the intestinal tract and ferment quickly, has been shown to significantly reduce symptoms of irritable bowel syndrome (IBS). This diet is based on the premise that certain carbohydrates can exacerbate the symptoms of IBS, including bloating, gas, and abdominal pain. By reducing the intake of these carbohydrates, many people find substantial relief from their symptoms, highlighting the critical role that diet plays in managing conditions like IBS.

Furthermore, dietary lipids have conflicting effects on the health of the digestive system. Although vitamin absorption and general health depend on good fats, consuming too much-saturated fat might worsen reflux disease (GERD) and other digestive problems. This is due to the fact that eating fatty meals may cause the lower esophageal sphincter to relax, enabling stomach acid to pass through and result in heartburn.

The diet also affects the acidity and enzyme activity within the digestive tract, which can influence how well nutrients are absorbed and how effectively the body can digest food. An imbalance can lead to discomfort, nutrient deficiencies, and increased susceptibility to digestive disorders. Thus, maintaining a balanced diet that includes a variety of nutrients can help ensure optimal enzyme and acid levels, promoting efficient digestion and absorption.

The LOW-FODMAP Diet: A Comprehensive Guide

Understanding the LOW-FODMAP Diet: A Lifesaver for Digestive Disorders

The LOW-FODMAP diet has emerged as a transformative approach for countless individuals grappling with chronic digestive disorders. This diet tackles the dietary causes of gut discomfort, with a particular emphasis on restricting foods high in fermentable oligosaccharides, disaccharides, monosaccharides, and polyols. For many, adopting this dietary regimen has brought about profound changes, offering not just relief from physical symptoms but also enhancing emotional well-being and overall quality of life.

One of the most immediate benefits reported by those following the LOW-FODMAP diet is the significant reduction in abdominal pain and bloating. These symptoms are often debilitating and can severely impact daily activities. By reducing the intake of FODMAPs, the diet minimizes the fermentation in the large intestine that typically leads to gas production and subsequent bloating and discomfort. For individuals who have lived with constant abdominal pain, this relief can feel miraculous, restoring their ability to engage in activities without the looming fear of pain.

Furthermore, the LOW-FODMAP diet has been particularly effective in managing irregular bowel habits, such as diarrhea and constipation, which are common among individuals with IBS and other functional gastrointestinal disorders. The diet helps stabilize the digestive system by eliminating foods that lead to rapid or delayed gastric emptying. As these individuals experience more regular bowel movements, their overall sense of health improves, allowing for a more active and engaged lifestyle.

Beyond the physical improvements, the diet also offers psychological benefits. Chronic digestive issues often carry a psychological toll, including increased anxiety and stress about when and where symptoms may occur. The predictability and control afforded by the LOW-FODMAP diet reduce this stress, giving individuals confidence in managing their condition. This psychological relief is profound as it impacts not just the individual but also their interactions with friends and family and their ability to participate in social activities.

The LOW-FODMAP diet also promotes a deeper understanding of one's body. Through the process of eliminating and reintroducing various foods, individuals become attuned to the specific triggers that exacerbate their symptoms. This knowledge empowers them to make informed dietary choices, which is crucial for long-term management of their condition. Being equipped with this knowledge transforms their approach to eating from one of caution and restriction to one of confident decision-making.

Moreover, the diet's structured approach to identifying food intolerances has broader health implications. For instance, many people discover intolerances they previously were unaware of, which may have contributed to other health issues beyond digestive symptoms, such as skin rashes, headaches, or fatigue. Addressing these intolerances can lead to an overall improvement in health and vitality, which might not have been achieved without following the structured elimination and reintroduction phases of the LOW-FODMAP diet.

Importantly, the LOW-FODMAP diet has fostered a supportive community of sufferers, healthcare providers, and dietitians, all focused on understanding and managing digestive health. This community provides a platform for sharing experiences, tips, and recipes, further easing the burden of managing a restrictive diet. The sense of community and shared experience reduces feelings of isolation and fosters a collective knowledge that benefits all members.

What are FODMAPs? Breaking Down the Acronym

FODMAPs, which stand for fermentable oligosaccharides, disaccharides, monosaccharides, and polyols, are phrases that have become more and more recognizable to people navigating the difficulties of digestive diseases. These little carbs and sugar alcohols are found in many different foods, such as grains, sweeteners, and fruits and vegetables. FODMAPs are widely consumed, but for some people, especially those with sensitive stomachs or diseases like Irritable Bowel Syndrome (IBS), they can cause severe digestive pain.

The component "Fermentable" in FODMAPs refers to the process by which gut bacteria ferment undigested carbohydrates to produce gas, a major contributor to bloating, pain, and other gastrointestinal symptoms associated with IBS. This fermentation process is a normal part of digestion but can become problematic in sensitive individuals.

"Oligosaccharides" are short-chain carbohydrates found in foods such as garlic, onions, wheat, and legumes. These substances are not absorbed by the small intestine, which means they pass through to the colon, where they are fermented by bacteria, leading to gas production and potentially contributing to the discomfort and bloating experienced by those with IBS.

Milk, soft cheeses, and yogurt are examples of dairy products that include "disaccharides," of which lactose is the most well-known. Lactase is an enzyme that breaks down lactose, and it is absent in those who are lactose intolerant. Consequently, undigested lactose passes into the colon, where it is fermented by bacteria, causing gas, bloating, and diarrhea.

"Monosaccharides," particularly fructose, present another challenge. High levels of fructose are found in honey, apples, and high-fructose corn syrup, among other foods. For individuals with fructose malabsorption, excess fructose is not adequately absorbed in the small intestine, similarly leading to fermentation in the colon and the accompanying symptoms of pain, gas, and bloating.

Finally, "Polyols," or sugar alcohols, are found in some fruits and vegetables like mushrooms and apricots, as well as in artificial sweeteners such as sorbitol and mannitol. Like other FODMAPs, these are poorly absorbed by the small intestine and thus fermented by bacteria in the colon, contributing to the array of digestive symptoms.

For those without digestive issues, FODMAPs generally do not pose problems and can be part of a healthy diet. However, for individuals with IBS or similar gastrointestinal sensitivities, FODMAPs can trigger symptoms severe enough to significantly impact quality of life. The reason these carbohydrates cause discomfort is not fully understood, but it is clear that their poor absorption in the small intestine leads to increased fluid and gas in the bowel, which then results in bloating, pain, and altered bowel movements.

The connection between FODMAPs and digestive distress led to the development of the LOW-FODMAP diet, a dietary approach that minimizes the intake of these fermentable carbohydrates. The diet has been clinically shown to reduce symptoms in a significant proportion of individuals with IBS. By limiting foods high in FODMAPs, the diet helps to decrease the amount of fermentable material available to gut bacteria, thereby reducing the fermentation process that causes gas and discomfort.

Benefits of a LOW-FODMAP Diet: Beyond Just Digestive Relief

The original goal of the LOW-FODMAP diet was to reduce the symptoms of Irritable Bowel Syndrome (IBS) and other gastrointestinal diseases. However, research has shown that there are a number of other health advantages to the diet that go well beyond just improving digestion. For many, following this diet not only diminishes the direct discomforts of digestion but also significantly enhances overall quality of life and general health.

One of the most significant advantages of adhering to a LOW-FODMAP diet is the notable improvement in energy levels. Individuals with digestive issues often experience fatigue and lethargy, partly due to the body's intense effort to deal with undigested food particles that ferment in the gut, leading to gas and bloating. The diet lessens these fermentation processes by consuming fewer FODMAPs, which lessens the strain on the body and increases the amount of energy available. People may have a more active lifestyle and participate in more everyday activities thanks to their increased energy, which improves their mental and physical health.

Improved sleep patterns are another notable benefit linked to the LOW-FODMAP diet. Digestive distress can significantly disrupt sleep due to discomfort and frequent trips to the bathroom. With the reduction in gastrointestinal symptoms, many find that their sleep quality improves, which is crucial for overall health. Better sleep not only helps in repairing and restoring the body but also improves mood, cognitive function, and stress management.

Furthermore, the diet's emphasis on the careful selection of foods can lead to a more nutritious diet overall. As individuals on a LOW-FODMAP diet become more mindful of the foods they consume, they often make healthier food choices, opting for a variety of low-FODMAP fruits, vegetables, grains, and proteins that are less likely to induce symptoms. This can lead to an increased intake of vitamins, minerals, and antioxidants, which play critical roles in overall health and disease prevention.

The psychological benefits of following a LOW-FODMAP diet should not be underestimated. Chronic digestive issues can have a profound impact on an individual’s mental health, often leading to or exacerbating conditions such as anxiety and depression. The diet's ability to reduce symptoms can result in notable gains in mental health. The reduction of constant worry about digestive discomfort allows individuals to feel more in control of their health, which is empowering and can significantly reduce stress and anxiety levels.

The LOW-FODMAP diet also often results in a healthier gut microbiome over time. Although initially, the reduction in certain carbohydrates might decrease the breadth of gut flora, many find that with careful reintroduction and balance, their gut flora adapts and may even improve. A healthy microbiome is crucial for digestion, immune function, and even mood regulation, as emerging research suggests a strong link between gut health and mental health.

Social well-being is another area where many see improvements. Digestive discomfort can be isolating, as it may deter individuals from social activities and gatherings, especially those involving food. As symptoms improve, confidence in participating in social events tends to increase, enhancing social interactions and support networks, which are vital components of overall happiness and life satisfaction.

BREAKFAST

Low-FODMAP Blueberry Banana Pancakes

Ingredients:

- 1 cup gluten-free flour
- 1 tablespoon sugar
- 1 teaspoon baking powder
- 1/2 teaspoon baking soda
- 1/4 teaspoon salt
- 1 cup lactose-free milk
- 1 egg
- 1 ripe banana, mashed
- 1/2 cup fresh blueberries
- 2 tablespoons vegetable oil

Directions:

1. In a large bowl, mix the gluten-free flour, sugar, baking powder, baking soda, and salt.
2. In another bowl, whisk together the lactose-free milk, egg, and mashed banana.
3. Pour the wet ingredients into the dry ingredients and stir until just combined. Gently fold in the blueberries.
4. Heat a non-stick skillet over medium heat and lightly grease it with vegetable oil.
5. Pour 1/4 cup of batter onto the skillet for each pancake. Cook until bubbles form on the surface, then flip and cook until golden brown.
6. Serve immediately.

Nutritional Values (per serving):

- Calories: 200
- Fat: 8g
- Carbohydrates: 30g
- Protein: 4g

Spinach and Feta Omelette

Ingredients:

- 2 eggs
- 1/4 cup fresh spinach, chopped
- 2 tablespoons feta cheese, crumbled
- Salt and pepper to taste
- 1 tablespoon olive oil

Directions:

1. In a bowl, beat the eggs with salt and pepper.
2. Heat olive oil in a non-stick skillet over medium heat.
3. Pour the eggs into the skillet and cook for about 1-2 minutes, until the edges start to set.
4. Sprinkle the chopped spinach and feta cheese over one half of the omelette.
5. Fold the omelette in half and cook for another minute, until the spinach is wilted and the cheese is melted.
6. Serve immediately.

Nutritional Values (per serving):

- Calories: 250
- Fat: 20g
- Carbohydrates: 2g
- Protein: 14g

Low-FODMAP Overnight Oats with Strawberries

Ingredients:

- 1/2 cup gluten-free oats
- 1/2 cup lactose-free milk
- 1/4 cup strawberries, sliced
- 1 tablespoon chia seeds
- 1 tablespoon maple syrup

Directions:

1. In a jar or container, combine the oats, lactose-free milk, chia seeds, and maple syrup.
2. Stir well, then top with sliced strawberries.
3. Cover and refrigerate overnight.
4. In the morning, stir the oats and enjoy.

Nutritional Values (per serving):

- Calories: 220
- Fat: 7g
- Carbohydrates: 35g
- Protein: 6g

Quinoa Porridge with Maple and Pecans

Ingredients:

- 1 cup cooked quinoa
- 1/2 cup lactose-free milk
- 1 tablespoon maple syrup
- 2 tablespoons chopped pecans
- 1/4 teaspoon cinnamon

Directions:

1. In a saucepan, combine the cooked quinoa, lactose-free milk, and cinnamon. Heat over medium heat until warmed through.
2. Stir in the maple syrup.

3. Divide the porridge into bowls and top with chopped pecans.
4. Serve immediately.

Nutritional Values (per serving):

- Calories: 300
- Fat: 12g
- Carbohydrates: 40g
- Protein: 8g

Low-FODMAP Avocado Toast on Gluten-Free Bread

Ingredients:

- 2 slices gluten-free bread
- 1 ripe avocado
- Salt and pepper to taste
- Optional toppings: cherry tomatoes, arugula, red pepper flakes

Directions:

1. Toast the gluten-free bread slices to your desired crispness.
2. Halve the avocado, remove the pit, and scoop the flesh into a bowl. Mash it with a fork and season with salt and pepper.
3. Spread the mashed avocado evenly on each slice of toasted bread.
4. Add optional toppings like sliced cherry tomatoes, arugula, or a sprinkle of red pepper flakes for extra flavor.
5. Serve immediately.

Nutritional Values (per serving):

- Calories: 280
- Fat: 18g
- Carbohydrates: 24g
- Protein: 4g

Scrambled Eggs with Spinach and Lactose-Free Cheese

Ingredients:

- 2 eggs
- 1/4 cup fresh spinach, chopped
- 1/4 cup lactose-free cheese, shredded
- Salt and pepper to taste
- 1 tablespoon olive oil

Directions:

1. In a bowl, beat the eggs with salt and pepper.
2. Heat olive oil in a non-stick skillet over medium heat.
3. Add the chopped spinach and cook until wilted.

4. Pour the eggs into the skillet and cook, stirring gently, until they start to set.
5. Add the shredded cheese and continue to cook until the eggs are fully set and the cheese is melted.
6. Serve immediately.

Nutritional Values (per serving):

- Calories: 250
- Fat: 20g
- Carbohydrates: 2g
- Protein: 14g

Rice Cakes with Peanut Butter and Banana Slices

Ingredients:

- 2 rice cakes
- 2 tablespoons peanut butter
- 1 banana, sliced

Directions:

1. Spread a tablespoon of peanut butter on each rice cake.
2. Top with banana slices.
3. Serve immediately.

Nutritional Values (per serving):

- Calories: 200
- Fat: 10g
- Carbohydrates: 25g
- Protein: 5g

Coconut Yogurt Parfait with Low-FODMAP Granola

Ingredients:

- 1 cup coconut yogurt
- 1/2 cup low-FODMAP granola
- 1/4 cup blueberries

Directions:

1. Layer the coconut yogurt, granola, and blueberries in a bowl or glass.
2. Serve immediately.

Nutritional Values (per serving):

- Calories: 300
- Fat: 15g
- Carbohydrates: 35g
- Protein: 6g

Low-FODMAP Smoothie Bowl with Kiwi and Pineapple

Ingredients:

- 1 cup lactose-free yogurt
- 1/2 cup frozen pineapple chunks
- 1 kiwi, peeled and sliced
- 1 tablespoon chia seeds
- 1/4 cup low-FODMAP granola

Directions:

1. Blend the lactose-free yogurt and frozen pineapple until smooth.
2. Pour into a bowl and top with sliced kiwi, chia seeds, and granola.
3. Serve immediately.

Nutritional Values (per serving):

- Calories: 350
- Fat: 12g
- Carbohydrates: 50g
- Protein: 10g

Oatmeal with Chia Seeds and Blueberries

Ingredients:

- 1/2 cup gluten-free oats
- 1 cup water or lactose-free milk
- 1 tablespoon chia seeds
- 1/4 cup blueberries
- 1 tablespoon maple syrup

Directions:

1. Combine oats and water or milk in a saucepan and bring to a boil.
2. Reduce heat and simmer for 5-7 minutes, stirring occasionally, until the oats are cooked.
3. Stir in chia seeds and maple syrup.
4. Top with blueberries and serve immediately.

Nutritional Values (per serving):

- Calories: 250
- Fat: 6g
- Carbohydrates: 45g
- Protein: 7g

Low-FODMAP Pumpkin Spice Muffins

Ingredients:

- 1 1/2 cups gluten-free flour
- 1 cup canned pumpkin
- 1/2 cup sugar
- 1/4 cup vegetable oil
- 2 eggs
- 1 teaspoon baking powder
- 1/2 teaspoon baking soda
- 1 teaspoon cinnamon
- 1/2 teaspoon nutmeg
- 1/4 teaspoon cloves
- 1/4 teaspoon salt

Directions:

1. Preheat oven to 350°F (175°C) and line a muffin tin with paper liners.
2. In a large bowl, combine the flour, baking powder, baking soda,

cinnamon, nutmeg, cloves, and salt.

3. In another bowl, mix the pumpkin, sugar, vegetable oil, and eggs until smooth.
4. Add the wet ingredients to the dry ingredients and stir until just combined.
5. Divide the batter evenly among the muffin cups.
6. Bake for 20-25 minutes, or until a toothpick inserted into the center comes out clean.
7. Cool on a wire rack and serve.

Nutritional Values (per serving):

- Calories: 180
- Fat: 8g
- Carbohydrates: 24g
- Protein: 3g

Poached Eggs on Gluten-Free Toast with Tomato Slices

Ingredients:

- 2 eggs
- 2 slices gluten-free bread
- 1 tomato, sliced
- Salt and pepper to taste
- 1 tablespoon vinegar

Directions:

1. Bring a pot of water to a gentle simmer and add vinegar.
2. Create a gentle whirlpool in the water, crack each egg into a small bowl, and gently tip them into the simmering water.
3. Cook for 3-4 minutes for soft poached eggs, or longer for firmer yolks.
4. Remove the eggs with a slotted spoon and set aside on a warm plate.
5. Toast the gluten-free bread slices.
6. Arrange tomato slices on the toast and top with poached eggs.
7. Season with salt and pepper and serve immediately.

Nutritional Values (per serving):

- Calories: 250
- Fat: 10g
- Carbohydrates: 28g
- Protein: 12g

Low-FODMAP Protein Pancakes with Maple Syrup

Ingredients:

- 1 cup gluten-free flour
- 1/4 cup protein powder

- 1 tablespoon sugar
- 1 teaspoon baking powder
- 1/2 teaspoon baking soda
- 1/4 teaspoon salt
- 1 cup lactose-free milk
- 1 egg
- 1 tablespoon vegetable oil
- Maple syrup for serving

Directions:

1. In a large bowl, mix the flour, protein powder, sugar, baking powder, baking soda, and salt.
2. In another bowl, whisk together the lactose-free milk, egg, and vegetable oil.
3. Pour the wet ingredients into the dry ingredients and stir until just combined.
4. Heat a non-stick skillet over medium heat and lightly grease with vegetable oil.
5. Pour 1/4 cup of batter onto the skillet for each pancake. Cook until bubbles form on the surface, then flip and cook until golden brown.
6. Serve with maple syrup.

Nutritional Values (per serving):

- Calories: 230
- Fat: 8g
- Carbohydrates: 30g
- Protein: 10g

Lactose-Free Cottage Cheese with Fresh Strawberries

Ingredients:

- 1 cup lactose-free cottage cheese
- 1/2 cup fresh strawberries, sliced

Directions:

1. Place the cottage cheese in a bowl.
2. Top with sliced strawberries.
3. Serve immediately.

Nutritional Values (per serving):

- Calories: 150
- Fat: 2g
- Carbohydrates: 14g
- Protein: 20g

Baked Sweet Potato with Almond Butter and Cinnamon

Ingredients:

- 1 medium sweet potato
- 1 tablespoon almond butter
- 1/4 teaspoon cinnamon

Directions:

1. Preheat oven to 400°F (200°C).
2. Pierce the sweet potato with a fork and bake for 45-60 minutes, until tender.
3. Cut the sweet potato open and top with almond butter and cinnamon.
4. Serve immediately.

Nutritional Values (per serving):

- Calories: 220
- Fat: 8g
- Carbohydrates: 35g
- Protein: 4g

Greek Yogurt with Low-FODMAP Fruit Compote

Ingredients:

- 1 cup lactose-free Greek yogurt
- 1/2 cup low-FODMAP fruit compote (e.g., strawberries, blueberries, or kiwi)
- 1 tablespoon honey (optional)

Directions:

1. Place the Greek yogurt in a bowl.
2. Top with low-FODMAP fruit compote.
3. Drizzle with honey if desired.
4. Serve immediately.

Nutritional Values (per serving):

- Calories: 180
- Fat: 5g
- Carbohydrates: 20g
- Protein: 15g

Spinach and Cheddar Frittata

Ingredients:

- 4 eggs
- 1/2 cup lactose-free cheddar cheese, shredded
- 1 cup fresh spinach, chopped
- Salt and pepper to taste
- 1 tablespoon olive oil

Directions:

1. Preheat oven to 350°F (175°C).
2. In a bowl, beat the eggs with salt and pepper.
3. Heat olive oil in an oven-safe skillet over medium heat.
4. Add the chopped spinach and cook until wilted.
5. Pour the beaten eggs into the skillet and cook for 2-3 minutes, until the edges start to set.
6. Sprinkle the shredded cheddar cheese on top.

7. Transfer the skillet to the oven and bake for 10-12 minutes, until the frittata is fully set.
8. Serve immediately.

Nutritional Values (per serving):

- Calories: 200
- Fat: 15g
- Carbohydrates: 2g
- Protein: 12g

Rice Porridge with Cinnamon and Maple Syrup

Ingredients:

- 1 cup cooked white rice
- 1 cup lactose-free milk
- 1 tablespoon maple syrup
- 1/2 teaspoon cinnamon

Directions:

1. In a saucepan, combine the cooked rice and lactose-free milk. Heat over medium heat until warmed through.
2. Stir in the maple syrup and cinnamon.
3. Serve immediately.

Nutritional Values (per serving):

- Calories: 220
- Fat: 4g
- Carbohydrates: 40g
- Protein: 5g

Low-FODMAP Banana Nut Muffins

Ingredients:

- 1 1/2 cups gluten-free flour
- 1/2 cup walnuts, chopped
- 1/2 cup sugar
- 1/4 cup vegetable oil
- 2 eggs
- 2 ripe bananas, mashed
- 1 teaspoon baking powder
- 1/2 teaspoon baking soda
- 1/4 teaspoon salt

Directions:

1. Preheat oven to 350°F (175°C) and line a muffin tin with paper liners.
2. In a large bowl, combine the flour, baking powder, baking soda, and salt.
3. In another bowl, mix the mashed bananas, sugar, vegetable oil, and eggs until smooth.
4. Add the wet ingredients to the dry ingredients and stir until just combined.
5. Fold in the chopped walnuts.

6. Divide the batter evenly among the muffin cups.
7. Bake for 20-25 minutes, or until a toothpick inserted into the center comes out clean.
8. Cool on a wire rack and serve.

Nutritional Values (per serving):

- Calories: 180
- Fat: 8g
- Carbohydrates: 25g
- Protein: 3g

Scrambled Tofu with Bell Peppers and Spinach

Ingredients:

- 1 block firm tofu, drained and crumbled
- 1/2 cup bell peppers, diced
- 1 cup fresh spinach, chopped
- 1 tablespoon olive oil
- 1/2 teaspoon turmeric
- Salt and pepper to taste

Directions:

1. Heat olive oil in a non-stick skillet over medium heat.
2. Add the diced bell peppers and cook until softened.
3. Add the crumbled tofu and turmeric, stirring to combine.
4. Cook for 5-7 minutes, until the tofu is heated through.
5. Add the chopped spinach and cook until wilted.
6. Season with salt and pepper.
7. Serve immediately.

Nutritional Values (per serving):

- Calories: 200
- Fat: 14g
- Carbohydrates: 6g
- Protein: 14g

LUNCH

Low-FODMAP Quinoa Salad with Roasted Vegetables

Ingredients:

- 1 cup quinoa
- 2 cups water
- 1 cup zucchini, diced
- 1 cup red bell pepper, diced
- 1 cup eggplant, diced
- 2 tablespoons olive oil
- Salt and pepper to taste
- 1/4 cup fresh parsley, chopped
- 1 tablespoon lemon juice

Directions:

1. Preheat oven to 400°F (200°C).
2. Toss zucchini, red bell pepper, and eggplant with olive oil, salt, and pepper. Spread on a baking sheet and roast for 20-25 minutes, until tender.
3. While vegetables are roasting, rinse quinoa under cold water. Combine quinoa and water in a pot, bring to a boil, then reduce heat and simmer for 15 minutes until water is absorbed and quinoa is fluffy.
4. In a large bowl, combine cooked quinoa, roasted vegetables, parsley, and lemon juice. Mix well.
5. Serve immediately.

Nutritional Values (per serving):

- Calories: 250
- Fat: 10g
- Carbohydrates: 35g
- Protein: 7g

Grilled Chicken and Spinach Wraps

Ingredients:

- 2 grilled chicken breasts, sliced
- 2 cups fresh spinach
- 4 gluten-free tortillas
- 1/4 cup lactose-free Greek yogurt
- 1 tablespoon Dijon mustard
- Salt and pepper to taste

Directions:

1. In a small bowl, mix Greek yogurt, Dijon mustard, salt, and pepper to make the dressing.
2. Lay out the tortillas and spread a tablespoon of the dressing on each.
3. Divide the grilled chicken and fresh spinach among the tortillas.
4. Roll up the tortillas tightly and serve immediately.

Nutritional Values (per serving):

- Calories: 300
- Fat: 8g
- Carbohydrates: 28g
- Protein: 30g

Low-FODMAP Tomato and Basil Soup

Ingredients:

- 4 large tomatoes, chopped
- 1 cup carrot, diced
- 1/4 cup fresh basil, chopped
- 2 cups low-FODMAP vegetable broth
- 2 tablespoons olive oil
- Salt and pepper to taste

Directions:

1. Heat olive oil in a large pot over medium heat. Add chopped tomatoes and carrots, cook for 10 minutes until softened.
2. Add the vegetable broth and bring to a boil. Reduce heat and simmer for 20 minutes.
3. Use an immersion blender to puree the soup until smooth.
4. Stir in chopped basil, season with salt and pepper.
5. Serve immediately.

Nutritional Values (per serving):

- Calories: 150
- Fat: 7g
- Carbohydrates: 20g
- Protein: 3g

Rice Noodle Salad with Shrimp and Cucumber

Ingredients:

- 8 oz rice noodles
- 1/2 lb cooked shrimp
- 1 cucumber, julienned
- 1/4 cup fresh mint, chopped
- 2 tablespoons lime juice
- 2 tablespoons fish sauce
- 1 tablespoon olive oil
- Salt and pepper to taste

Directions:

1. Cook rice noodles according to package instructions, then rinse under cold water and drain.

2. In a large bowl, combine rice noodles, shrimp, cucumber, and mint.
3. In a small bowl, whisk together lime juice, fish sauce, olive oil, salt, and pepper.
4. Pour the dressing over the salad and toss to combine.
5. Serve immediately.

Nutritional Values (per serving):

- Calories: 300
- Fat: 8g
- Carbohydrates: 40g
- Protein: 20g

Gluten-Free Turkey Club Sandwich

Ingredients:

- 4 slices gluten-free bread
- 4 oz sliced turkey breast
- 2 slices cooked bacon
- 1 tomato, sliced
- 2 leaves lettuce
- 2 tablespoons mayonnaise

Directions:

1. Toast the gluten-free bread slices.
2. Spread mayonnaise on each slice of bread.
3. Layer the turkey, bacon, tomato, and lettuce on two slices of bread, then top with the remaining bread slices.
4. Cut the sandwiches in half and serve immediately.

Nutritional Values (per serving):

- Calories: 400
- Fat: 18g
- Carbohydrates: 30g
- Protein: 25g

Low-FODMAP Greek Salad with Feta and Olives

Ingredients:

- 1 cup cherry tomatoes, halved
- 1 cucumber, diced
- 1/4 cup Kalamata olives, pitted and halved
- 1/4 cup feta cheese, crumbled
- 2 tablespoons olive oil
- 1 tablespoon lemon juice
- 1 teaspoon dried oregano
- Salt and pepper to taste

Directions:

1. In a large bowl, combine cherry tomatoes, cucumber, olives, and feta cheese.

2. In a small bowl, whisk together olive oil, lemon juice, oregano, salt, and pepper.
3. Pour the dressing over the salad and toss to combine.
4. Serve immediately.

Nutritional Values (per serving):

- Calories: 200
- Fat: 16g
- Carbohydrates: 10g
- Protein: 6g

Grilled Salmon with Quinoa and Asparagus

Ingredients:

- 2 salmon fillets
- 1 cup quinoa
- 2 cups water
- 1 bunch asparagus, trimmed
- 2 tablespoons olive oil
- 1 tablespoon lemon juice
- Salt and pepper to taste

Directions:

1. Preheat grill to medium-high heat.
2. Season salmon fillets with salt and pepper. Grill for 4-5 minutes on each side, until cooked through.
3. Rinse quinoa under cold water. Combine quinoa and water in a pot, bring to a boil, then reduce heat and simmer for 15 minutes until water is absorbed and quinoa is fluffy.
4. Toss asparagus with olive oil, salt, and pepper. Grill for 5-7 minutes until tender.
5. Serve grilled salmon with quinoa and asparagus, drizzled with lemon juice.

Nutritional Values (per serving):

- Calories: 450
- Fat: 20g
- Carbohydrates: 30g
- Protein: 35g

Low-FODMAP Stuffed Bell Peppers with Ground Turkey

Ingredients:

- 4 bell peppers, tops cut off and seeds removed
- 1 lb ground turkey
- 1 cup cooked rice
- 1 cup diced tomatoes
- 1/4 cup lactose-free cheese, shredded
- 1 tablespoon olive oil
- Salt and pepper to taste

Directions:

1. Preheat oven to 375°F (190°C).
2. Heat olive oil in a skillet over medium heat. Add ground turkey and cook until browned.
3. Stir in cooked rice and diced tomatoes, season with salt and pepper.
4. Stuff the bell peppers with the turkey mixture and place in a baking dish.
5. Top with shredded cheese and bake for 25-30 minutes, until peppers are tender and cheese is melted.
6. Serve immediately.

Nutritional Values (per serving):

- Calories: 300
- Fat: 12g
- Carbohydrates: 20g
- Protein: 25g

Chicken Caesar Salad (Low-FODMAP Dressing)

Ingredients:

- 2 grilled chicken breasts, sliced
- 4 cups romaine lettuce, chopped
- 1/4 cup lactose-free Parmesan cheese, shredded
- 1/2 cup gluten-free croutons

Low-FODMAP Dressing:

- 1/4 cup lactose-free Greek yogurt
- 1 tablespoon olive oil
- 1 tablespoon lemon juice
- 1 teaspoon Dijon mustard
- 1 clove garlic-infused olive oil
- Salt and pepper to taste

Directions:

1. In a small bowl, whisk together Greek yogurt, olive oil, lemon juice, Dijon mustard, garlic-infused olive oil, salt, and pepper.
2. In a large bowl, combine romaine lettuce, grilled chicken, Parmesan cheese, and croutons.
3. Drizzle with dressing and toss to combine.
4. Serve immediately.

Nutritional Values (per serving):

- Calories: 350
- Fat: 18g
- Carbohydrates: 15g
- Protein: 30g

Sweet Potato and Zucchini Fritters

Ingredients:

- 1 cup grated sweet potato
- 1 cup grated zucchini
- 1 egg
- 1/4 cup gluten-free flour
- 2 tablespoons olive oil
- Salt and pepper to taste

Directions:

1. In a large bowl, combine grated sweet potato, zucchini, egg, gluten-free flour, salt, and pepper.
2. Heat olive oil in a non-stick skillet over medium heat.
3. Spoon 1/4 cup of the mixture into the skillet, flattening it into a fritter shape. Cook for 3-4 minutes on each side until golden brown and crispy.
4. Repeat with the remaining mixture.
5. Serve immediately.

Nutritional Values (per serving):

- Calories: 200
- Fat: 12g
- Carbohydrates: 18g
- Protein: 4g

Low-FODMAP Lentil Soup with Spinach

Ingredients:

- 1 cup green lentils
- 4 cups low-FODMAP vegetable broth
- 1 cup carrots, diced
- 1 cup celery, diced
- 2 cups fresh spinach, chopped
- 2 tablespoons olive oil
- Salt and pepper to taste

Directions:

1. Heat olive oil in a large pot over medium heat. Add carrots and celery, cook until softened.
2. Add lentils and vegetable broth, bring to a boil. Reduce heat and simmer for 30 minutes until lentils are tender.
3. Stir in chopped spinach, season with salt and pepper.
4. Serve immediately.

Nutritional Values (per serving):

- Calories: 250
- Fat: 8g
- Carbohydrates: 35g
- Protein: 12g

Baked Cod with Quinoa and Roasted Carrots

Ingredients:

- 2 cod fillets
- 1 cup quinoa
- 2 cups water
- 2 cups carrots, sliced
- 2 tablespoons olive oil
- 1 tablespoon lemon juice
- Salt and pepper to taste

Directions:

1. Preheat oven to 375°F (190°C).
2. Season cod fillets with salt and pepper, place on a baking sheet.
3. Toss sliced carrots with olive oil, salt, and pepper. Spread on a separate baking sheet.
4. Bake cod and carrots for 20-25 minutes until fish is cooked through and carrots are tender.
5. Rinse quinoa under cold water. Combine quinoa and water in a pot, bring to a boil, then reduce heat and simmer for 15 minutes until water is absorbed and quinoa is fluffy.
6. Serve baked cod with quinoa and roasted carrots, drizzled with lemon juice.

Nutritional Values (per serving):

- Calories: 400
- Fat: 14g
- Carbohydrates: 35g
- Protein: 30g

Low-FODMAP Tofu Stir-Fry with Bok Choy

Ingredients:

- 1 block firm tofu, drained and cubed
- 2 cups bok choy, chopped
- 1 red bell pepper, sliced
- 2 tablespoons sesame oil
- 2 tablespoons low-sodium soy sauce
- 1 tablespoon ginger, grated
- 1 tablespoon garlic-infused olive oil

Directions:

1. Heat sesame oil in a large skillet over medium-high heat.
2. Add cubed tofu and cook until golden brown on all sides. Remove from skillet and set aside.
3. In the same skillet, add garlic-infused olive oil, grated ginger, bok choy, and red bell pepper. Cook until vegetables are tender.

4. Return tofu to the skillet, add soy sauce, and stir to combine.
5. Serve immediately.

Nutritional Values (per serving):

- Calories: 250
- Fat: 16g
- Carbohydrates: 10g
- Protein: 14g

Grilled Chicken Salad with Strawberries and Almonds

Ingredients:

- 2 grilled chicken breasts, sliced
- 4 cups mixed greens
- 1 cup strawberries, sliced
- 1/4 cup almonds, sliced
- 2 tablespoons olive oil
- 1 tablespoon balsamic vinegar
- Salt and pepper to taste

Directions:

1. In a large bowl, combine mixed greens, grilled chicken, strawberries, and almonds.
2. In a small bowl, whisk together olive oil, balsamic vinegar, salt, and pepper.
3. Drizzle the dressing over the salad and toss to combine.
4. Serve immediately.

Nutritional Values (per serving):

- Calories: 350
- Fat: 20g
- Carbohydrates: 15g
- Protein: 30g

Low-FODMAP Pasta Salad with Roasted Vegetables

Ingredients:

- 8 oz gluten-free pasta
- 1 cup zucchini, diced
- 1 cup cherry tomatoes, halved
- 1 red bell pepper, diced
- 2 tablespoons olive oil
- 1/4 cup fresh basil, chopped
- 2 tablespoons balsamic vinegar
- Salt and pepper to taste

Directions:

1. Preheat oven to 400°F (200°C).
2. Toss zucchini, cherry tomatoes, and red bell pepper with olive oil, salt, and pepper. Spread on a baking sheet and roast for 20-25 minutes until tender.
3. Cook gluten-free pasta according to package instructions, then drain and rinse under cold water.
4. In a large bowl, combine cooked pasta, roasted vegetables, fresh

basil, and balsamic vinegar. Toss to combine.

5. Serve immediately.

Nutritional Values (per serving):

- Calories: 300
- Fat: 12g
- Carbohydrates: 40g
- Protein: 6g

Turkey and Swiss Lettuce Wraps

Ingredients:

- 8 slices turkey breast
- 4 leaves large lettuce
- 4 slices Swiss cheese
- 1/4 cup mayonnaise
- 1 tablespoon Dijon mustard

Directions:

1. In a small bowl, mix mayonnaise and Dijon mustard.
2. Lay out the lettuce leaves and spread the mayonnaise mixture on each.
3. Place two slices of turkey and one slice of Swiss cheese on each lettuce leaf.
4. Roll up the lettuce wraps and serve immediately.

Nutritional Values (per serving):

- Calories: 250
- Fat: 18g
- Carbohydrates: 2g
- Protein: 20g

Low-FODMAP Thai Chicken Salad

Ingredients:

- 2 grilled chicken breasts, sliced
- 4 cups mixed greens
- 1/2 cup shredded carrots
- 1/2 cup cucumber, julienned
- 1/4 cup fresh cilantro, chopped
- 2 tablespoons lime juice
- 2 tablespoons fish sauce
- 1 tablespoon olive oil
- Salt and pepper to taste

Directions:

1. In a large bowl, combine mixed greens, grilled chicken, shredded carrots, cucumber, and cilantro.
2. In a small bowl, whisk together lime juice, fish sauce, olive oil, salt, and pepper.
3. Drizzle the dressing over the salad and toss to combine.
4. Serve immediately.

Nutritional Values (per serving):

- Calories: 300
- Fat: 15g
- Carbohydrates: 10g
- Protein: 30g

Baked Tilapia with Lemon and Dill

Ingredients:

- 2 tilapia fillets
- 1 tablespoon olive oil
- 1 tablespoon lemon juice
- 1 teaspoon dried dill
- Salt and pepper to taste

Directions:

1. Preheat oven to 375°F (190°C).
2. Place tilapia fillets on a baking sheet and drizzle with olive oil and lemon juice.
3. Sprinkle with dried dill, salt, and pepper.
4. Bake for 15-20 minutes until fish is cooked through and flakes easily with a fork.
5. Serve immediately.

Nutritional Values (per serving):

- Calories: 200
- Fat: 10g
- Carbohydrates: 1g
- Protein: 25g

Quinoa and Roasted Beet Salad

Ingredients:

- 1 cup quinoa
- 2 cups water
- 2 medium beets, roasted and diced
- 1/4 cup feta cheese, crumbled
- 1/4 cup fresh parsley, chopped
- 2 tablespoons olive oil
- 1 tablespoon balsamic vinegar
- Salt and pepper to taste

Directions:

1. Preheat oven to 400°F (200°C). Wrap beets in foil and roast for 45-60 minutes until tender. Let cool, peel, and dice.
2. Rinse quinoa under cold water. Combine quinoa and water in a pot, bring to a boil, then reduce heat and simmer for 15 minutes until water is absorbed and quinoa is fluffy.
3. In a large bowl, combine cooked quinoa, roasted beets, feta cheese, and parsley.
4. In a small bowl, whisk together olive oil, balsamic vinegar, salt, and pepper.

5. Pour the dressing over the salad and toss to combine.
6. Serve immediately.

Nutritional Values (per serving):

- Calories: 300
- Fat: 12g
- Carbohydrates: 40g
- Protein: 8g

Low-FODMAP Chicken and Rice Soup

Ingredients:

- 1 lb chicken breasts, diced
- 1 cup carrots, diced
- 1 cup celery, diced
- 1/2 cup long grain rice
- 6 cups low-FODMAP chicken broth
- 2 tablespoons olive oil
- Salt and pepper to taste

Directions:

1. Heat olive oil in a large pot over medium heat. Add diced chicken and cook until browned.
2. Add carrots and celery, cook until softened.
3. Stir in rice and chicken broth. Bring to a boil, then reduce heat and simmer for 20 minutes until rice is cooked.
4. Season with salt and pepper.
5. Serve immediately.

Nutritional Values (per serving):

- Calories: 300
- Fat: 10g
- Carbohydrates: 25g
- Protein: 25g

Grilled Vegetable and Hummus Sandwich

Ingredients:

- 1 zucchini, sliced
- 1 red bell pepper, sliced
- 1 eggplant, sliced
- 4 slices gluten-free bread
- 1/2 cup low-FODMAP hummus
- 2 tablespoons olive oil
- Salt and pepper to taste

Directions:

1. Preheat grill to medium-high heat.
2. Toss zucchini, red bell pepper, and eggplant slices with olive oil, salt, and pepper. Grill until tender.
3. Toast the gluten-free bread slices.
4. Spread hummus on each slice of bread.

5. Layer grilled vegetables on two slices of bread, then top with the remaining slices.
6. Serve immediately.

Nutritional Values (per serving):

- Calories: 350
- Fat: 18g
- Carbohydrates: 40g
- Protein: 8g

Low-FODMAP Chicken and Avocado Salad

Ingredients:

- 2 grilled chicken breasts, sliced
- 1 avocado, diced
- 4 cups mixed greens
- 1/4 cup cherry tomatoes, halved
- 2 tablespoons olive oil
- 1 tablespoon lemon juice
- Salt and pepper to taste

Directions:

1. In a large bowl, combine mixed greens, grilled chicken, avocado, and cherry tomatoes.
2. In a small bowl, whisk together olive oil, lemon juice, salt, and pepper.
3. Drizzle the dressing over the salad and toss to combine.
4. Serve immediately.

Nutritional Values (per serving):

- Calories: 400
- Fat: 25g
- Carbohydrates: 12g
- Protein: 30g

Rice Paper Rolls with Shrimp and Cucumber

Ingredients:

- 8 rice paper sheets
- 1/2 lb cooked shrimp
- 1 cucumber, julienned
- 1/4 cup fresh mint, chopped
- 1/4 cup fresh cilantro, chopped
- 1/4 cup carrots, julienned
- 2 tablespoons rice vinegar

Directions:

1. Dip rice paper sheets in warm water to soften, then lay them flat on a clean surface.
2. Arrange shrimp, cucumber, mint, cilantro, and carrots in the center of each sheet.
3. Drizzle with rice vinegar.
4. Roll up each sheet tightly, folding in the sides as you go.
5. Serve immediately.

Nutritional Values (per serving):

- Calories: 150
- Fat: 1g
- Carbohydrates: 20g
- Protein: 15g

Tuna Salad with Gluten-Free Crackers

Ingredients:

- 1 can tuna, drained
- 2 tablespoons mayonnaise
- 1 tablespoon Dijon mustard
- 1 tablespoon fresh parsley, chopped
- Salt and pepper to taste
- Gluten-free crackers

Directions:

1. In a bowl, combine tuna, mayonnaise, Dijon mustard, parsley, salt, and pepper.
2. Mix well.
3. Serve with gluten-free crackers.

Nutritional Values (per serving):

- Calories: 200
- Fat: 10g
- Carbohydrates: 15g
- Protein: 15g

Low-FODMAP Chickpea Salad with Lemon Dressing

Ingredients:

- 1 can chickpeas, drained and rinsed
- 1 cup cucumber, diced
- 1 cup cherry tomatoes, halved
- 1/4 cup fresh parsley, chopped
- 2 tablespoons olive oil
- 1 tablespoon lemon juice
- Salt and pepper to taste

Directions:

1. In a large bowl, combine chickpeas, cucumber, cherry tomatoes, and parsley.
2. In a small bowl, whisk together olive oil, lemon juice, salt, and pepper.
3. Pour the dressing over the salad and toss to combine.
4. Serve immediately.

Nutritional Values (per serving):

- Calories: 250
- Fat: 12g
- Carbohydrates: 30g
- Protein: 8g

DINNER

Grilled Lemon Herb Chicken with Quinoa

Ingredients:

- 2 boneless, skinless chicken breasts
- 1 cup quinoa
- 2 cups water
- 2 tablespoons olive oil
- 1 tablespoon lemon juice
- 1 teaspoon dried oregano
- 1 teaspoon dried thyme
- Salt and pepper to taste

Directions:

1. In a small bowl, mix olive oil, lemon juice, oregano, thyme, salt, and pepper. Marinate the chicken breasts in this mixture for at least 30 minutes.
2. Preheat grill to medium-high heat. Grill the chicken for 6-7 minutes on each side, or until fully cooked.
3. Rinse quinoa under cold water. Combine quinoa and water in a pot, bring to a boil, then reduce heat and simmer for 15 minutes until water is absorbed and quinoa is fluffy.
4. Serve grilled chicken over quinoa.

Nutritional Values (per serving):

- Calories: 400
- Fat: 14g
- Carbohydrates: 30g
- Protein: 35g

Low-FODMAP Baked Salmon with Dill and Green Beans

Ingredients:

- 2 salmon fillets
- 2 cups green beans, trimmed
- 2 tablespoons olive oil
- 1 tablespoon fresh dill, chopped
- 1 tablespoon lemon juice
- Salt and pepper to taste

Directions:

1. Preheat oven to 375°F (190°C).
2. Place salmon fillets on a baking sheet. Drizzle with olive oil and lemon juice, then sprinkle with dill, salt, and pepper.

3. Toss green beans with olive oil, salt, and pepper. Arrange them around the salmon on the baking sheet.
4. Bake for 20-25 minutes, until salmon is cooked through and green beans are tender.
5. Serve immediately.

Nutritional Values (per serving):

- Calories: 350
- Fat: 18g
- Carbohydrates: 10g
- Protein: 35g

Beef Stir-Fry with Bok Choy and Carrots

Ingredients:

- 1 lb beef sirloin, thinly sliced
- 2 cups bok choy, chopped
- 1 cup carrots, julienned
- 2 tablespoons sesame oil
- 2 tablespoons low-sodium soy sauce
- 1 tablespoon garlic-infused olive oil
- 1 tablespoon ginger, grated
- Salt and pepper to taste

Directions:

1. Heat sesame oil in a large skillet over medium-high heat.
2. Add beef slices and cook until browned. Remove from skillet and set aside.
3. In the same skillet, add garlic-infused olive oil, grated ginger, bok choy, and carrots. Cook until vegetables are tender.
4. Return beef to the skillet, add soy sauce, and stir to combine.
5. Serve immediately.

Nutritional Values (per serving):

- Calories: 300
- Fat: 18g
- Carbohydrates: 10g
- Protein: 25g

Low-FODMAP Chicken Alfredo with Gluten-Free Pasta

Ingredients:

- 2 chicken breasts, diced
- 8 oz gluten-free pasta
- 1 cup lactose-free cream
- 1/2 cup lactose-free Parmesan cheese, grated
- 2 tablespoons olive oil

- 1 tablespoon garlic-infused olive oil
- Salt and pepper to taste

Directions:

1. Cook gluten-free pasta according to package instructions, then drain and set aside.
2. Heat olive oil in a skillet over medium heat. Add diced chicken and cook until browned and fully cooked.
3. In a saucepan, heat lactose-free cream over medium heat. Stir in garlic-infused olive oil and grated Parmesan cheese, cooking until cheese is melted and sauce is thickened.
4. Combine cooked pasta, chicken, and Alfredo sauce. Mix well.
5. Serve immediately.

Nutritional Values (per serving):

- Calories: 450
- Fat: 20g
- Carbohydrates: 40g
- Protein: 30g

Stuffed Bell Peppers with Quinoa and Ground Beef

Ingredients:

- 4 bell peppers, tops cut off and seeds removed
- 1 lb ground beef
- 1 cup cooked quinoa
- 1 cup diced tomatoes
- 1/4 cup lactose-free cheese, shredded
- 2 tablespoons olive oil
- Salt and pepper to taste

Directions:

1. Preheat oven to 375°F (190°C).
2. Heat olive oil in a skillet over medium heat. Add ground beef and cook until browned.
3. Stir in cooked quinoa and diced tomatoes, season with salt and pepper.
4. Stuff the bell peppers with the beef mixture and place in a baking dish.
5. Top with shredded cheese and bake for 25-30 minutes, until peppers are tender and cheese is melted.
6. Serve immediately.

Nutritional Values (per serving):

- Calories: 350
- Fat: 18g
- Carbohydrates: 20g
- Protein: 30g

Low-FODMAP Shrimp and Vegetable Skewers

Ingredients:

- 1 lb shrimp, peeled and deveined
- 1 zucchini, sliced
- 1 red bell pepper, diced
- 1 cup cherry tomatoes
- 2 tablespoons olive oil
- 1 tablespoon lemon juice
- Salt and pepper to taste

Directions:

1. Preheat grill to medium-high heat.
2. In a large bowl, combine shrimp, zucchini, red bell pepper, and cherry tomatoes. Toss with olive oil, lemon juice, salt, and pepper.
3. Thread the shrimp and vegetables onto skewers.
4. Grill for 2-3 minutes on each side, until shrimp is cooked through and vegetables are tender.
5. Serve immediately.

Nutritional Values (per serving):

- Calories: 250
- Fat: 10g
- Carbohydrates: 10g
- Protein: 30g

Baked Chicken Thighs with Sweet Potatoes

Ingredients:

- 4 chicken thighs
- 2 large sweet potatoes, peeled and diced
- 2 tablespoons olive oil
- 1 tablespoon rosemary, chopped
- Salt and pepper to taste

Directions:

1. Preheat oven to 375°F (190°C).
2. Toss sweet potatoes with olive oil, rosemary, salt, and pepper. Spread on a baking sheet.
3. Season chicken thighs with salt and pepper and place them on top of the sweet potatoes.
4. Bake for 35-40 minutes, until chicken is cooked through and sweet potatoes are tender.
5. Serve immediately.

Nutritional Values (per serving):

- Calories: 400
- Fat: 20g
- Carbohydrates: 30g
- Protein: 25g

Low-FODMAP Vegetable Curry with Tofu

Ingredients:

- 1 block firm tofu, drained and cubed
- 2 cups carrots, sliced
- 2 cups green beans, trimmed
- 1 can coconut milk
- 2 tablespoons curry powder
- 1 tablespoon olive oil
- Salt and pepper to taste

Directions:

1. Heat olive oil in a large skillet over medium heat. Add cubed tofu and cook until golden brown.
2. Add carrots and green beans, cooking until tender.
3. Stir in coconut milk and curry powder, bringing to a simmer. Cook for 10 minutes, until vegetables are fully cooked.
4. Season with salt and pepper.
5. Serve immediately.

Nutritional Values (per serving):

- Calories: 300
- Fat: 20g
- Carbohydrates: 20g
- Protein: 12g

Roasted Turkey Breast with Low-FODMAP Gravy

Ingredients:

- 1 turkey breast
- 2 tablespoons olive oil
- 1 tablespoon fresh thyme, chopped
- 1 cup low-FODMAP chicken broth
- 1 tablespoon cornstarch
- Salt and pepper to taste

Directions:

1. Preheat oven to 375°F (190°C).
2. Rub turkey breast with olive oil, thyme, salt, and pepper. Place in a roasting pan.
3. Roast for 45-60 minutes, until turkey is cooked through.
4. In a saucepan, heat chicken broth over medium heat. Stir in cornstarch, cooking until thickened.
5. Serve turkey breast with gravy.

Nutritional Values (per serving):

- Calories: 350
- Fat: 15g
- Carbohydrates: 5g
- Protein: 45g

Low-FODMAP Shepherd's Pie with Sweet Potato Topping

Ingredients:

- 1 lb ground beef
- 2 cups carrots, diced
- 2 cups green beans, trimmed
- 2 large sweet potatoes, peeled and mashed
- 1 cup low-FODMAP beef broth
- 2 tablespoons olive oil
- Salt and pepper to taste

Directions:

1. Preheat oven to 375°F (190°C).
2. Heat olive oil in a skillet over medium heat. Add ground beef and cook until browned.
3. Stir in carrots, green beans, and beef broth. Simmer until vegetables are tender.
4. Transfer beef mixture to a baking dish. Spread mashed sweet potatoes over the top.
5. Bake for 25-30 minutes, until topping is golden brown.
6. Serve immediately.

Nutritional Values (per serving):

- Calories: 400
- Fat: 18g
- Carbohydrates: 30g
- Protein: 25g

Grilled Pork Chops with Quinoa and Green Beans

Ingredients:

- 2 pork chops
- 1 cup quinoa
- 2 cups water
- 2 cups green beans, trimmed
- 2 tablespoons olive oil
- 1 tablespoon lemon juice
- Salt and pepper to taste

Directions:

1. Preheat grill to medium-high heat. Season pork chops with salt and pepper.
2. Grill pork chops for 6-7 minutes on each side, until fully cooked.
3. Rinse quinoa under cold water. Combine quinoa and water in a pot, bring to a boil, then reduce heat and simmer for 15 minutes until water is absorbed and quinoa is fluffy.
4. Steam green beans until tender.
5. Serve grilled pork chops with quinoa and green beans, drizzled with lemon juice.

Nutritional Values (per serving):

- Calories: 450
- Fat: 20g
- Carbohydrates: 30g
- Protein: 35g

Low-FODMAP Eggplant Parmesan

Ingredients:

- 1 large eggplant, sliced
- 1 cup gluten-free breadcrumbs
- 1/2 cup lactose-free Parmesan cheese, grated
- 2 eggs, beaten
- 2 cups low-FODMAP marinara sauce
- 2 tablespoons olive oil
- Salt and pepper to taste

Directions:

1. Preheat oven to 375°F (190°C). Line a baking sheet with parchment paper.
2. Dip eggplant slices in beaten eggs, then coat with gluten-free breadcrumbs mixed with Parmesan cheese.
3. Place coated eggplant slices on the baking sheet and drizzle with olive oil.
4. Bake for 20-25 minutes until golden brown.
5. In a baking dish, layer baked eggplant slices with marinara sauce and remaining Parmesan cheese.
6. Bake for an additional 15 minutes until cheese is melted and bubbly.
7. Serve immediately.

Nutritional Values (per serving):

- Calories: 300
- Fat: 15g
- Carbohydrates: 30g
- Protein: 10g

Lemon Garlic Shrimp with Zucchini Noodles

Ingredients:

- 1 lb shrimp, peeled and deveined
- 2 zucchinis, spiralized into noodles
- 2 tablespoons olive oil
- 1 tablespoon lemon juice
- 1 tablespoon garlic-infused olive oil
- Salt and pepper to taste

Directions:

1. Heat olive oil in a large skillet over medium heat. Add shrimp and cook until pink and opaque.

2. Add garlic-infused olive oil, lemon juice, salt, and pepper. Stir to combine.
3. Add zucchini noodles to the skillet and cook for 2-3 minutes until tender.
4. Serve immediately.

Nutritional Values (per serving):

- Calories: 250
- Fat: 12g
- Carbohydrates: 10g
- Protein: 25g

Low-FODMAP Beef and Broccoli Stir-Fry

Ingredients:

- 1 lb beef sirloin, thinly sliced
- 2 cups broccoli florets
- 1/4 cup low-sodium soy sauce
- 2 tablespoons garlic-infused olive oil
- 1 tablespoon ginger, grated
- 2 tablespoons sesame oil
- Salt and pepper to taste

Directions:

1. Heat sesame oil in a large skillet over medium-high heat.
2. Add beef slices and cook until browned. Remove from skillet and set aside.
3. In the same skillet, add garlic-infused olive oil, grated ginger, and broccoli florets. Cook until broccoli is tender.
4. Return beef to the skillet, add soy sauce, and stir to combine.
5. Serve immediately.

Nutritional Values (per serving):

- Calories: 300
- Fat: 18g
- Carbohydrates: 10g
- Protein: 25g

Baked Cod with Lemon and Roasted Asparagus

Ingredients:

- 2 cod fillets
- 1 bunch asparagus, trimmed
- 2 tablespoons olive oil
- 1 tablespoon lemon juice
- Salt and pepper to taste

Directions:

1. Preheat oven to 375°F (190°C).
2. Place cod fillets on a baking sheet. Drizzle with olive oil and lemon juice, then season with salt and pepper.

3. Toss asparagus with olive oil, salt, and pepper. Arrange around the cod on the baking sheet.
4. Bake for 20-25 minutes, until cod is cooked through and asparagus is tender.
5. Serve immediately.

Nutritional Values (per serving):

- Calories: 250
- Fat: 10g
- Carbohydrates: 5g
- Protein: 30g

Low-FODMAP Chicken and Rice Casserole

Ingredients:

- 2 chicken breasts, diced
- 1 cup long grain rice
- 2 cups low-FODMAP chicken broth
- 1 cup carrots, diced
- 1 cup green beans, trimmed
- 2 tablespoons olive oil
- Salt and pepper to taste

Directions:

1. Preheat oven to 375°F (190°C).
2. Heat olive oil in a skillet over medium heat. Add diced chicken and cook until browned.
3. In a baking dish, combine chicken, rice, chicken broth, carrots, and green beans. Season with salt and pepper.
4. Cover with foil and bake for 45-50 minutes until rice is tender and liquid is absorbed.
5. Serve immediately.

Nutritional Values (per serving):

- Calories: 350
- Fat: 10g
- Carbohydrates: 40g
- Protein: 25g

Grilled Lamb Chops with Quinoa Salad

Ingredients:

- 4 lamb chops
- 1 cup quinoa
- 2 cups water
- 1 cup cherry tomatoes, halved
- 1/4 cup fresh mint, chopped
- 2 tablespoons olive oil
- 1 tablespoon lemon juice
- Salt and pepper to taste

Directions:

1. Preheat grill to medium-high heat. Season lamb chops with salt and pepper.

2. Grill lamb chops for 4-5 minutes on each side, until desired doneness.
3. Rinse quinoa under cold water. Combine quinoa and water in a pot, bring to a boil, then reduce heat and simmer for 15 minutes until water is absorbed and quinoa is fluffy.
4. In a large bowl, combine cooked quinoa, cherry tomatoes, fresh mint, olive oil, lemon juice, salt, and pepper.
5. Serve grilled lamb chops with quinoa salad.

Nutritional Values (per serving):

- Calories: 450
- Fat: 25g
- Carbohydrates: 30g
- Protein: 30g

Low-FODMAP Stuffed Acorn Squash with Quinoa

Ingredients:

- 2 acorn squashes, halved and seeded
- 1 cup quinoa
- 2 cups water
- 1/4 cup dried cranberries
- 1/4 cup walnuts, chopped
- 2 tablespoons olive oil
- 1 tablespoon maple syrup
- Salt and pepper to taste

Directions:

1. Preheat oven to 375°F (190°C). Place acorn squash halves on a baking sheet and drizzle with olive oil. Roast for 35-40 minutes until tender.
2. Rinse quinoa under cold water. Combine quinoa and water in a pot, bring to a boil, then reduce heat and simmer for 15 minutes until water is absorbed and quinoa is fluffy.
3. In a large bowl, combine cooked quinoa, dried cranberries, walnuts, olive oil, maple syrup, salt, and pepper.
4. Stuff the roasted acorn squash halves with the quinoa mixture.
5. Serve immediately.

Nutritional Values (per serving):

- Calories: 350
- Fat: 15g
- Carbohydrates: 45g
- Protein: 8g

Baked Chicken Breasts with Lemon and Rosemary

Ingredients:

- 2 chicken breasts
- 2 tablespoons olive oil
- 1 tablespoon lemon juice
- 1 tablespoon fresh rosemary, chopped
- Salt and pepper to taste

Directions:

1. Preheat oven to 375°F (190°C).
2. Rub chicken breasts with olive oil, lemon juice, rosemary, salt, and pepper. Place in a baking dish.
3. Bake for 25-30 minutes until chicken is cooked through.
4. Serve immediately.

Nutritional Values (per serving):

- Calories: 300
- Fat: 15g
- Carbohydrates: 2g
- Protein: 35g

Low-FODMAP Mushroom Risotto

Ingredients:

- 1 cup Arborio rice
- 4 cups low-FODMAP chicken broth
- 1 cup mushrooms, sliced
- 1/2 cup lactose-free Parmesan cheese, grated
- 2 tablespoons olive oil
- 1 tablespoon garlic-infused olive oil
- Salt and pepper to taste

Directions:

1. Heat olive oil and garlic-infused olive oil in a large skillet over medium heat. Add mushrooms and cook until tender.
2. Stir in Arborio rice and cook for 1-2 minutes until slightly toasted.
3. Gradually add chicken broth, one cup at a time, stirring constantly until the liquid is absorbed before adding more.
4. Continue until the rice is tender and creamy.
5. Stir in grated Parmesan cheese, salt, and pepper.
6. Serve immediately.

Nutritional Values (per serving):

- Calories: 350
- Fat: 12g
- Carbohydrates: 50g
- Protein: 10g

Grilled Salmon with Low-FODMAP Pesto and Vegetables

Ingredients:

- 2 salmon fillets
- 2 cups mixed vegetables (zucchini, bell peppers, cherry tomatoes)
- 2 tablespoons olive oil
- 1/4 cup low-FODMAP pesto
- Salt and pepper to taste

Directions:

1. Preheat grill to medium-high heat.
2. Toss mixed vegetables with olive oil, salt, and pepper. Grill until tender.
3. Season salmon fillets with salt and pepper. Grill for 4-5 minutes on each side until cooked through.
4. Serve grilled salmon with grilled vegetables and a dollop of low-FODMAP pesto.

Nutritional Values (per serving):

- Calories: 400
- Fat: 25g
- Carbohydrates: 10g
- Protein: 30g

Low-FODMAP Tofu and Vegetable Stir-Fry

Ingredients:

- 1 block firm tofu, drained and cubed
- 2 cups mixed vegetables (bell peppers, broccoli, carrots)
- 2 tablespoons sesame oil
- 2 tablespoons low-sodium soy sauce
- 1 tablespoon garlic-infused olive oil
- 1 tablespoon ginger, grated
- Salt and pepper to taste

Directions:

1. Heat sesame oil in a large skillet over medium-high heat.
2. Add cubed tofu and cook until golden brown. Remove from skillet and set aside.
3. In the same skillet, add garlic-infused olive oil, grated ginger, and mixed vegetables. Cook until vegetables are tender.
4. Return tofu to the skillet, add soy sauce, and stir to combine.
5. Serve immediately.

Nutritional Values (per serving):

- Calories: 250
- Fat: 16g
- Carbohydrates: 10g
- Protein: 14g

Baked Tilapia with Roasted Brussels Sprouts

Ingredients:

- 2 tilapia fillets
- 2 cups Brussels sprouts, halved
- 2 tablespoons olive oil
- 1 tablespoon lemon juice
- Salt and pepper to taste

Directions:

1. Preheat oven to 375°F (190°C).
2. Place tilapia fillets on a baking sheet. Drizzle with olive oil and lemon juice, then season with salt and pepper.
3. Toss Brussels sprouts with olive oil, salt, and pepper. Arrange around the tilapia on the baking sheet.
4. Bake for 20-25 minutes, until tilapia is cooked through and Brussels sprouts are tender.
5. Serve immediately.

Nutritional Values (per serving):

- Calories: 250
- Fat: 10g
- Carbohydrates: 10g
- Protein: 30g

Low-FODMAP Chicken Tacos with Corn Tortillas

Ingredients:

- 2 chicken breasts, diced
- 8 corn tortillas
- 1 cup shredded lettuce
- 1/2 cup lactose-free cheese, shredded
- 1/4 cup salsa (ensure low-FODMAP ingredients)
- 2 tablespoons olive oil
- Salt and pepper to taste

Directions:

1. Heat olive oil in a skillet over medium heat. Add diced chicken and cook until browned and fully cooked.
2. Warm corn tortillas in a dry skillet or microwave.
3. Divide cooked chicken among tortillas, then top with shredded lettuce, cheese, and salsa.
4. Serve immediately.

Nutritional Values (per serving):

- Calories: 300
- Fat: 12g
- Carbohydrates: 20g
- Protein: 25g

Grilled Vegetable Kebabs with Quinoa

Ingredients:

- 1 zucchini, sliced
- 1 red bell pepper, diced
- 1 yellow bell pepper, diced
- 1 red onion, cut into chunks
- 1 cup cherry tomatoes
- 1 cup quinoa
- 2 cups water
- 2 tablespoons olive oil
- 1 tablespoon balsamic vinegar
- Salt and pepper to taste

Directions:

1. Preheat grill to medium-high heat.
2. Thread zucchini, bell peppers, red onion, and cherry tomatoes onto skewers. Brush with olive oil and season with salt and pepper.
3. Grill vegetable kebabs for 10-12 minutes, turning occasionally, until vegetables are tender and slightly charred.
4. Rinse quinoa under cold water. Combine quinoa and water in a pot, bring to a boil, then reduce heat and simmer for 15 minutes until water is absorbed and quinoa is fluffy.
5. In a large bowl, toss cooked quinoa with balsamic vinegar, salt, and pepper.
6. Serve grilled vegetable kebabs over quinoa.

Nutritional Values (per serving):

- Calories: 350
- Fat: 14g
- Carbohydrates: 40g
- Protein: 8g

Scan the QR Code and access your 3 bonuses in digital format

🔥 Bonus 1: 60 Day Meal Plan

🔥 Bonus 2: Emotional Well-being Tips

🔥 Bonus 3: Low Fodmap grocery shopping list

SNACKS

Low-FODMAP Almond Butter Energy Balls

Ingredients:

- 1 cup gluten-free rolled oats
- 1/2 cup almond butter
- 1/4 cup maple syrup
- 1/4 cup unsweetened shredded coconut
- 1 tablespoon chia seeds

Directions:

1. In a large bowl, combine all ingredients and mix well.
2. Roll the mixture into small balls, about 1 inch in diameter.
3. Place the energy balls on a baking sheet lined with parchment paper and refrigerate for at least 30 minutes.
4. Store in an airtight container in the refrigerator.

Nutritional Values (per serving):

- Calories: 150
- Fat: 9g
- Carbohydrates: 15g
- Protein: 4g

Rice Cakes with Lactose-Free Cottage Cheese and Cucumber

Ingredients:

- 2 rice cakes
- 1/2 cup lactose-free cottage cheese
- 1/2 cucumber, thinly sliced
- Salt and pepper to taste

Directions:

1. Spread lactose-free cottage cheese on each rice cake.
2. Top with thinly sliced cucumber.
3. Season with salt and pepper.
4. Serve immediately.

Nutritional Values (per serving):

- Calories: 120
- Fat: 2g
- Carbohydrates: 18g
- Protein: 6g

Low-FODMAP Trail Mix with Almonds and Dark Chocolate

Ingredients:

- 1/2 cup almonds
- 1/2 cup dark chocolate chips (ensure low-FODMAP)
- 1/4 cup pumpkin seeds
- 1/4 cup dried cranberries (ensure low-FODMAP)

Directions:

1. In a bowl, combine almonds, dark chocolate chips, pumpkin seeds, and dried cranberries.
2. Mix well and store in an airtight container.

Nutritional Values (per serving):

- Calories: 200
- Fat: 14g
- Carbohydrates: 18g
- Protein: 5g

Gluten-Free Crackers with Low-FODMAP Hummus

Ingredients:

- 1 cup low-FODMAP hummus
- Gluten-free crackers

Directions:

1. Serve low-FODMAP hummus in a bowl.
2. Accompany with gluten-free crackers.
3. Serve immediately.

Nutritional Values (per serving):

- Calories: 180
- Fat: 8g
- Carbohydrates: 20g
- Protein: 5g

Low-FODMAP Pumpkin Seed Granola Bars

Ingredients:

- 1 cup gluten-free rolled oats
- 1/2 cup pumpkin seeds
- 1/4 cup maple syrup
- 1/4 cup almond butter
- 1/4 cup dried cranberries (ensure low-FODMAP)

Directions:

1. Preheat oven to 350°F (175°C). Line a baking dish with parchment paper.
2. In a large bowl, combine all ingredients and mix well.
3. Press the mixture into the baking dish.

4. Bake for 20-25 minutes until golden brown.
5. Let cool, then cut into bars.
6. Store in an airtight container.

Nutritional Values (per serving):

- Calories: 200
- Fat: 10g
- Carbohydrates: 25g
- Protein: 5g

Lactose-Free Yogurt with Blueberries

Ingredients:

- 1 cup lactose-free yogurt
- 1/4 cup fresh blueberries

Directions:

1. Place lactose-free yogurt in a bowl.
2. Top with fresh blueberries.
3. Serve immediately.

Nutritional Values (per serving):

- Calories: 150
- Fat: 2g
- Carbohydrates: 22g
- Protein: 8g

Sliced Cucumber with Low-FODMAP Ranch Dip

Ingredients:

- 1 cucumber, sliced
- 1/2 cup lactose-free Greek yogurt
- 1 tablespoon fresh dill, chopped
- 1 tablespoon fresh chives, chopped
- 1 teaspoon garlic-infused olive oil
- Salt and pepper to taste

Directions:

1. In a bowl, combine lactose-free Greek yogurt, fresh dill, fresh chives, garlic-infused olive oil, salt, and pepper.
2. Mix well to create the ranch dip.
3. Serve sliced cucumber with the ranch dip.

Nutritional Values (per serving):

- Calories: 100
- Fat: 3g
- Carbohydrates: 12g
- Protein: 5g

Low-FODMAP Peanut Butter and Banana Rice Cakes

Ingredients:

- 2 rice cakes
- 2 tablespoons peanut butter

- 1 banana, sliced

Directions:

1. Spread a tablespoon of peanut butter on each rice cake.
2. Top with banana slices.
3. Serve immediately.

Nutritional Values (per serving):

- Calories: 200
- Fat: 10g
- Carbohydrates: 25g
- Protein: 5g

Low-FODMAP Smoothie with Spinach and Pineapple

Ingredients:

- 1 cup lactose-free yogurt
- 1/2 cup frozen pineapple chunks
- 1/2 cup fresh spinach
- 1 tablespoon chia seeds

Directions:

1. Blend lactose-free yogurt, frozen pineapple, fresh spinach, and chia seeds until smooth.
2. Pour into a glass and serve immediately.

Nutritional Values (per serving):

- Calories: 180
- Fat: 5g
- Carbohydrates: 25g
- Protein: 8g

Low-FODMAP Apple Slices with Almond Butter

Ingredients:

- 1 apple, sliced
- 2 tablespoons almond butter

Directions:

1. Slice the apple.
2. Serve apple slices with almond butter for dipping.
3. Serve immediately.

Nutritional Values (per serving):

- Calories: 180
- Fat: 10g
- Carbohydrates: 20g
- Protein: 4g

Gluten-Free Pretzels with Low-FODMAP Guacamole

Ingredients:

- 1 cup gluten-free pretzels
- 1 avocado
- 1 tablespoon lime juice
- 1 tablespoon fresh cilantro, chopped
- Salt and pepper to taste

Directions:

1. In a bowl, mash avocado with lime juice, fresh cilantro, salt, and pepper to make guacamole.
2. Serve gluten-free pretzels with guacamole.
3. Serve immediately.

Nutritional Values (per serving):

- Calories: 200
- Fat: 12g
- Carbohydrates: 20g
- Protein: 3g

Low-FODMAP Cheese and Grapes

Ingredients:

- 1/2 cup lactose-free cheese, cubed
- 1/2 cup grapes

Directions:

1. Arrange lactose-free cheese cubes and grapes on a plate.
2. Serve immediately.

Nutritional Values (per serving):

- Calories: 150
- Fat: 8g
- Carbohydrates: 15g
- Protein: 6g

Low-FODMAP Chia Pudding with Berries

Ingredients:

- 1/4 cup chia seeds
- 1 cup lactose-free milk
- 1 tablespoon maple syrup
- 1/2 cup fresh berries (ensure low-FODMAP)

Directions:

1. In a bowl, combine chia seeds, lactose-free milk, and maple syrup.
2. Mix well and refrigerate for at least 4 hours or overnight.
3. Top with fresh berries before serving.

Nutritional Values (per serving):

- Calories: 200
- Fat: 10g
- Carbohydrates: 25g
- Protein: 5g

Carrot Sticks with Low-FODMAP Hummus

Ingredients:

- 2 large carrots, peeled and cut into sticks
- 1 cup low-FODMAP hummus

Directions:

1. Arrange carrot sticks on a plate.
2. Serve with low-FODMAP hummus.

Nutritional Values (per serving):

- Calories: 150
- Fat: 7g
- Carbohydrates: 18g
- Protein: 5g

Low-FODMAP Celery Sticks with Peanut Butter

Ingredients:

- 2 celery stalks, cut into sticks
- 2 tablespoons peanut butter

Directions:

1. Spread peanut butter onto celery sticks.
2. Serve immediately.

Nutritional Values (per serving):

- Calories: 180
- Fat: 12g
- Carbohydrates: 12g
- Protein: 6g

DESSERTS

Low-FODMAP Blueberry Coconut Chia Pudding

Ingredients:

- 1/4 cup chia seeds
- 1 cup coconut milk
- 1 tablespoon maple syrup
- 1/2 cup fresh blueberries

Directions:

1. In a bowl, combine chia seeds, coconut milk, and maple syrup.
2. Mix well and refrigerate for at least 4 hours or overnight.
3. Top with fresh blueberries before serving.

Nutritional Values (per serving):

- Calories: 220
- Fat: 15g
- Carbohydrates: 20g
- Protein: 5g

Gluten-Free Chocolate Chip Cookies

Ingredients:

- 1 1/4 cups gluten-free flour
- 1/2 teaspoon baking soda
- 1/4 teaspoon salt
- 1/2 cup unsalted butter, softened
- 1/2 cup brown sugar
- 1/4 cup granulated sugar
- 1 large egg
- 1 teaspoon vanilla extract
- 1 cup dark chocolate chips (ensure low-FODMAP)

Directions:

1. Preheat oven to 350°F (175°C) and line a baking sheet with parchment paper.
2. In a bowl, whisk together gluten-free flour, baking soda, and salt.
3. In another bowl, cream together the butter, brown sugar, and granulated sugar until light and fluffy.
4. Beat in the egg and vanilla extract.
5. Gradually add the dry ingredients to the wet ingredients and mix until combined.
6. Fold in the chocolate chips.

7. Drop spoon fuls of dough onto the prepared baking sheet.
8. Bake for 10-12 minutes until the edges are golden.
9. Cool on a wire rack and serve.

Nutritional Values (per serving):

- Calories: 150
- Fat: 8g
- Carbohydrates: 20g
- Protein: 2g

Low-FODMAP Banana Bread

Ingredients:

- 1 1/2 cups gluten-free flour
- 1 teaspoon baking soda
- 1/4 teaspoon salt
- 3 ripe bananas, mashed
- 1/2 cup unsalted butter, melted
- 1/2 cup brown sugar
- 2 large eggs
- 1 teaspoon vanilla extract

Directions:

1. Preheat oven to 350°F (175°C) and grease a loaf pan.
2. In a bowl, whisk together gluten-free flour, baking soda, and salt.
3. In another bowl, mix together mashed bananas, melted butter, brown sugar, eggs, and vanilla extract.
4. Gradually add the dry ingredients to the wet ingredients and mix until just combined.
5. Pour the batter into the prepared loaf pan.
6. Bake for 60-70 minutes until a toothpick inserted into the center comes out clean.
7. Cool in the pan for 10 minutes, then transfer to a wire rack to cool completely.

Nutritional Values (per serving):

- Calories: 200
- Fat: 8g
- Carbohydrates: 30g
- Protein: 3g

Lactose-Free Cheesecake with a Gluten-Free Crust

Ingredients:

- 1 1/2 cups gluten-free graham cracker crumbs
- 1/4 cup unsalted butter, melted
- 2 cups lactose-free cream cheese, softened
- 1 cup granulated sugar
- 3 large eggs
- 1 teaspoon vanilla extract

Directions:

1. Preheat oven to 325°F (165°C) and grease a springform pan.
2. In a bowl, mix gluten-free graham cracker crumbs and melted butter. Press into the bottom of the prepared pan.
3. In another bowl, beat together lactose-free cream cheese and sugar until smooth.
4. Add eggs one at a time, beating well after each addition. Stir in vanilla extract.
5. Pour the cream cheese mixture over the crust.
6. Bake for 50-60 minutes until the center is set.
7. Cool in the pan, then refrigerate for at least 4 hours before serving.

Nutritional Values (per serving):

- Calories: 300
- Fat: 20g
- Carbohydrates: 28g
- Protein: 6g

Low-FODMAP Chocolate Avocado Mousse

Ingredients:

- 2 ripe avocados
- 1/4 cup unsweetened cocoa powder
- 1/4 cup maple syrup
- 1 teaspoon vanilla extract
- Pinch of salt

Directions:

1. In a food processor, blend avocados, cocoa powder, maple syrup, vanilla extract, and salt until smooth.
2. Spoon the mousse into serving bowls.
3. Refrigerate for at least 30 minutes before serving.

Nutritional Values (per serving):

- Calories: 250
- Fat: 18g
- Carbohydrates: 25g
- Protein: 3g

Low-FODMAP Carrot Cake with Cream Cheese Frosting

Ingredients:

- 1 1/2 cups gluten-free flour
- 1 teaspoon baking soda
- 1/2 teaspoon cinnamon
- 1/4 teaspoon nutmeg
- 1/4 teaspoon salt
- 3/4 cup granulated sugar
- 1/2 cup vegetable oil

- 2 large eggs
- 1 teaspoon vanilla extract
- 1 1/2 cups grated carrots
- 1/2 cup walnuts, chopped (optional)

Frosting:

- 1 cup lactose-free cream cheese, softened
- 1/4 cup unsalted butter, softened
- 2 cups powdered sugar
- 1 teaspoon vanilla extract

Directions:

1. Preheat oven to 350°F (175°C) and grease a 9-inch round cake pan.
2. In a bowl, whisk together gluten-free flour, baking soda, cinnamon, nutmeg, and salt.
3. In another bowl, mix together sugar, vegetable oil, eggs, and vanilla extract.
4. Gradually add the dry ingredients to the wet ingredients and mix until just combined.
5. Fold in grated carrots and walnuts.
6. Pour the batter into the prepared pan.
7. Bake for 30-35 minutes until a toothpick inserted into the center comes out clean.
8. Cool in the pan for 10 minutes, then transfer to a wire rack to cool completely.
9. For the frosting, beat together lactose-free cream cheese, butter, powdered sugar, and vanilla extract until smooth.
10. Spread the frosting over the cooled cake.

Nutritional Values (per serving):

- Calories: 350
- Fat: 18g
- Carbohydrates: 45g
- Protein: 4g

Strawberry Sorbet

Ingredients:

- 4 cups fresh strawberries, hulled
- 1/2 cup granulated sugar
- 1/2 cup water
- 1 tablespoon lemon juice

Directions:

1. In a blender, combine strawberries, sugar, water, and lemon juice. Blend until smooth.
2. Pour the mixture into an ice cream maker and freeze according to the manufacturer's instructions.
3. Serve immediately or store in the freezer.

Nutritional Values (per serving):

- Calories: 100
- Fat: 0g
- Carbohydrates: 25g
- Protein: 1g

Low-FODMAP Rice Pudding with Coconut Milk

Ingredients:

- 1 cup cooked white rice
- 2 cups coconut milk
- 1/4 cup maple syrup
- 1 teaspoon vanilla extract
- 1/4 teaspoon cinnamon

Directions:

1. In a saucepan, combine cooked rice, coconut milk, maple syrup, vanilla extract, and cinnamon.
2. Cook over medium heat, stirring frequently, until the mixture thickens, about 20 minutes.
3. Serve warm or chilled.

Nutritional Values (per serving):

- Calories: 250
- Fat: 10g
- Carbohydrates: 35g
- Protein: 3g

Gluten-Free Lemon Bars

Ingredients:

- 1 cup gluten-free flour
- 1/4 cup powdered sugar
- 1/2 cup unsalted butter, softened
- 1 cup granulated sugar
- 2 large eggs
- 1/4 cup lemon juice
- 1 teaspoon lemon zest

Directions:

1. Preheat oven to 350°F (175°C) and grease an 8-inch square baking dish.
2. In a bowl, mix together gluten-free flour, powdered sugar, and butter until crumbly. Press into the bottom of the prepared dish.
3. Bake for 15-20 minutes until lightly golden.
4. In another bowl, whisk together granulated sugar, eggs, lemon juice, and lemon zest.
5. Pour the lemon mixture over the baked crust.
6. Bake for an additional 20-25 minutes until set.
7. Cool completely, then cut into squares.

Nutritional Values (per serving):

- Calories: 200
- Fat: 10g
- Carbohydrates: 28g
- Protein: 2g

Low-FODMAP Apple Crisp

Ingredients:

- 4 cups peeled and sliced apples (ensure low-FODMAP variety)
- 1/2 cup gluten-free rolled oats
- 1/2 cup gluten-free flour
- 1/4 cup brown sugar
- 1/4 cup unsalted butter, melted
- 1 teaspoon cinnamon

Directions:

1. Preheat oven to 350°F (175°C) and grease a baking dish.
2. In a bowl, combine sliced apples and cinnamon. Place in the prepared baking dish.
3. In another bowl, mix together rolled oats, gluten-free flour, brown sugar, and melted butter until crumbly.
4. Sprinkle the oat mixture over the apples.
5. Bake for 30-35 minutes until the topping is golden and the apples are tender.
6. Serve warm.

Nutritional Values (per serving):

- Calories: 250
- Fat: 10g
- Carbohydrates: 40g
- Protein: 2g

Dark Chocolate Covered Strawberries

Ingredients:

- 1 cup dark chocolate chips (ensure low-FODMAP)
- 1 tablespoon coconut oil
- 1 pint fresh strawberries

Directions:

1. In a microwave-safe bowl, combine dark chocolate chips and coconut oil. Microwave in 30-second intervals, stirring until smooth.
2. Dip each strawberry into the melted chocolate, allowing the excess to drip off.
3. Place the strawberries on a baking sheet lined with parchment paper.
4. Refrigerate until the chocolate is set, about 30 minutes.

Nutritional Values (per serving):

- Calories: 150
- Fat: 10g

- Carbohydrates: 20g
- Protein: 1g

Low-FODMAP Mango Coconut Ice Cream

Ingredients:

- 2 ripe mangoes, peeled and diced
- 1 cup coconut milk
- 1/4 cup maple syrup
- 1 teaspoon vanilla extract

Directions:

1. In a blender, combine mangoes, coconut milk, maple syrup, and vanilla extract. Blend until smooth.
2. Pour the mixture into an ice cream maker and freeze according to the manufacturer's instructions.
3. Serve immediately or store in the freezer.

Nutritional Values (per serving):

- Calories: 180
- Fat: 8g
- Carbohydrates: 28g
- Protein: 1g

Gluten-Free Brownies

Ingredients:

- 1/2 cup unsalted butter, melted
- 1 cup granulated sugar
- 2 large eggs
- 1 teaspoon vanilla extract
- 1/3 cup gluten-free cocoa powder
- 1/2 cup gluten-free flour
- 1/4 teaspoon salt
- 1/4 teaspoon baking powder

Directions:

1. Preheat oven to 350°F (175°C) and grease an 8-inch square baking dish.
2. In a bowl, mix together melted butter, sugar, eggs, and vanilla extract.
3. Add cocoa powder, gluten-free flour, salt, and baking powder. Mix until well combined.
4. Pour the batter into the prepared dish.
5. Bake for 20-25 minutes until a toothpick inserted into the center comes out clean.
6. Cool completely, then cut into squares.

Nutritional Values (per serving):

- Calories: 180
- Fat: 8g
- Carbohydrates: 26g
- Protein: 2g

Low-FODMAP Cinnamon Sugar Donuts

Ingredients:

- 1 1/2 cups gluten-free flour
- 1/2 cup granulated sugar
- 1 teaspoon baking powder
- 1/2 teaspoon baking soda
- 1/2 teaspoon cinnamon
- 1/4 teaspoon salt
- 1/2 cup lactose-free milk
- 1/4 cup vegetable oil
- 2 large eggs
- 1 teaspoon vanilla extract
- 1/4 cup unsalted butter, melted (for coating)
- 1/2 cup granulated sugar (for coating)
- 1 teaspoon cinnamon (for coating)

Directions:

1. Preheat oven to 350°F (175°C) and grease a donut pan.
2. In a bowl, whisk together gluten-free flour, sugar, baking powder, baking soda, cinnamon, and salt.
3. In another bowl, mix together lactose-free milk, vegetable oil, eggs, and vanilla extract.
4. Gradually add the dry ingredients to the wet ingredients and mix until just combined.
5. Pour the batter into the prepared donut pan.
6. Bake for 12-15 minutes until a toothpick inserted into the center comes out clean.
7. Cool slightly, then brush with melted butter and coat with cinnamon sugar mixture.

Nutritional Values (per serving):

- Calories: 200
- Fat: 10g
- Carbohydrates: 25g
- Protein: 3g

Low-FODMAP Peach Cobbler with Almond Flour Crust

Ingredients:

- 4 cups sliced peaches (ensure low-FODMAP variety)
- 1/4 cup granulated sugar
- 1 teaspoon lemon juice
- 1/2 teaspoon cinnamon
- 1 cup almond flour
- 1/4 cup gluten-free flour
- 1/4 cup brown sugar

- 1/4 cup unsalted butter, melted
- 1/4 teaspoon salt

Directions:

1. Preheat oven to 350°F (175°C) and grease a baking dish.
2. In a bowl, combine sliced peaches, granulated sugar, lemon juice, and cinnamon. Place in the prepared baking dish.
3. In another bowl, mix together almond flour, gluten-free flour, brown sugar, melted butter, and salt until crumbly.
4. Sprinkle the crumb mixture over the peaches.
5. Bake for 30-35 minutes until the topping is golden and the peaches are tender.
6. Serve warm.

Nutritional Values (per serving):

- Calories: 250
- Fat: 12g
- Carbohydrates: 30g
- Protein: 4g

BONUS

60 Day Meal Plan (tables)

Days 1-10

Day	Breakfast	Lunch	Dinner	Snack
Day 1	Low-FODMAP Blueberry Banana Pancakes	Grilled Chicken and Spinach Wraps	Grilled Lemon Herb Chicken with Quinoa	Low-FODMAP Almond Butter Energy Balls
Day 2	Spinach and Feta Omelette	Low-FODMAP Tomato and Basil Soup	Low-FODMAP Baked Salmon with Dill and Green Beans	Rice Cakes with Peanut Butter and Banana Slices
Day 3	Low-FODMAP Overnight Oats with Strawberries	Rice Noodle Salad with Shrimp and Cucumber	Beef Stir-Fry with Bok Choy and Carrots	Lactose-Free Yogurt with Blueberries
Day 4	Quinoa Porridge with Maple and Pecans	Gluten-Free Turkey Club Sandwich	Low-FODMAP Chicken Alfredo with Gluten-Free Pasta	Sliced Cucumber with Low-FODMAP Ranch Dip
Day 5	Low-FODMAP Avocado Toast on Gluten-Free Bread	Low-FODMAP Greek Salad with Feta and Olives	Stuffed Bell Peppers with Quinoa and Ground Beef	Low-FODMAP Trail Mix with Almonds and Dark Chocolate

Day	Breakfast	Lunch	Dinner	Snack
Day 6	Scrambled Eggs with Spinach and Lactose-Free Cheese	Grilled Salmon with Quinoa and Asparagus	Low-FODMAP Shrimp and Vegetable Skewers	Gluten-Free Crackers with Low-FODMAP Hummus
Day 7	Rice Cakes with Peanut Butter and Banana Slices	Low-FODMAP Lentil Soup with Spinach	Baked Chicken Thighs with Sweet Potatoes	Low-FODMAP Pumpkin Seed Granola Bars
Day 8	Coconut Yogurt Parfait with Low-FODMAP Granola	Baked Cod with Quinoa and Roasted Carrots	Low-FODMAP Vegetable Curry with Tofu	Lactose-Free Cheese and Grapes
Day 9	Low-FODMAP Smoothie Bowl with Kiwi and Pineapple	Low-FODMAP Tofu Stir-Fry with Bok Choy	Roasted Turkey Breast with Low-FODMAP Gravy	Sliced Cucumber with Low-FODMAP Ranch Dip
Day 10	Oatmeal with Chia Seeds and Blueberries	Grilled Chicken Salad with Strawberries and Almonds	Low-FODMAP Shepherd's Pie with Sweet Potato Topping	Low-FODMAP Chia Pudding with Berries

Days 11-20

Day	Breakfast	Lunch	Dinner	Snack
Day 11	Low-FODMAP Pumpkin Spice Muffins	Low-FODMAP Pasta Salad with Roasted Vegetables	Grilled Pork Chops with Quinoa and Green Beans	Low-FODMAP Apple Slices with Almond Butter
Day 12	Poached Eggs on Gluten-Free Toast with Tomato Slices	Turkey and Swiss Lettuce Wraps	Low-FODMAP Eggplant Parmesan	Gluten-Free Pretzels with Low-FODMAP Guacamole
Day 13	Low-FODMAP Protein Pancakes with Maple Syrup	Low-FODMAP Thai Chicken Salad	Lemon Garlic Shrimp with Zucchini Noodles	Dark Chocolate Covered Strawberries
Day 14	Lactose-Free Cottage Cheese with Fresh Strawberries	Baked Tilapia with Lemon and Dill	Low-FODMAP Beef and Broccoli Stir-Fry	Carrot Sticks with Low-FODMAP Hummus
Day 15	Baked Sweet Potato with Almond Butter and Cinnamon	Quinoa and Roasted Beet Salad	Baked Cod with Lemon and Roasted Asparagus	Low-FODMAP Celery Sticks with Peanut Butter
Day 16	Greek Yogurt with Low-FODMAP Fruit Compote	Low-FODMAP Chicken and Rice Soup	Low-FODMAP Chicken and Rice Casserole	Low-FODMAP Almond Butter Energy Balls

Day	Breakfast	Lunch	Dinner	Snack
Day 17	Spinach and Cheddar Frittata	Grilled Vegetable and Hummus Sandwich	Grilled Lamb Chops with Quinoa Salad	Rice Cakes with Peanut Butter and Banana Slices
Day 18	Rice Porridge with Cinnamon and Maple Syrup	Low-FODMAP Chicken and Avocado Salad	Low-FODMAP Stuffed Acorn Squash with Quinoa	Lactose-Free Yogurt with Blueberries
Day 19	Low-FODMAP Banana Nut Muffins	Rice Paper Rolls with Shrimp and Cucumber	Baked Chicken Breasts with Lemon and Rosemary	Sliced Cucumber with Low-FODMAP Ranch Dip
Day 20	Scrambled Tofu with Bell Peppers and Spinach	Tuna Salad with Gluten-Free Crackers	Low-FODMAP Mushroom Risotto	Low-FODMAP Trail Mix with Almonds and Dark Chocolate

Days 21-30

Day	Breakfast	Lunch	Dinner	Snack
Day 21	Low-FODMAP Blueberry Banana Pancakes	Grilled Chicken and Spinach Wraps	Grilled Lemon Herb Chicken with Quinoa	Low-FODMAP Pumpkin Seed Granola Bars
Day 22	Spinach and Feta Omelette	Low-FODMAP Tomato and Basil Soup	Low-FODMAP Baked Salmon	Lactose-Free Cheese and Grapes

Day	Breakfast	Lunch	Dinner	Snack
			with Dill and Green Beans	
Day 23	Low-FODMAP Overnight Oats with Strawberries	Rice Noodle Salad with Shrimp and Cucumber	Beef Stir-Fry with Bok Choy and Carrots	Low-FODMAP Chia Pudding with Berries
Day 24	Quinoa Porridge with Maple and Pecans	Gluten-Free Turkey Club Sandwich	Low-FODMAP Chicken Alfredo with Gluten-Free Pasta	Dark Chocolate Covered Strawberries
Day 25	Low-FODMAP Avocado Toast on Gluten-Free Bread	Low-FODMAP Greek Salad with Feta and Olives	Stuffed Bell Peppers with Quinoa and Ground Beef	Low-FODMAP Almond Butter Energy Balls
Day 26	Scrambled Eggs with Spinach and Lactose-Free Cheese	Grilled Salmon with Quinoa and Asparagus	Low-FODMAP Shrimp and Vegetable Skewers	Low-FODMAP Apple Slices with Almond Butter
Day 27	Rice Cakes with Peanut Butter and Banana Slices	Low-FODMAP Lentil Soup with Spinach	Baked Chicken Thighs with Sweet Potatoes	Carrot Sticks with Low-FODMAP Hummus
Day 28	Coconut Yogurt Parfait with Low-FODMAP Granola	Baked Cod with Quinoa and Roasted Carrots	Low-FODMAP Vegetable Curry with Tofu	Gluten-Free Pretzels with Low-FODMAP Guacamole

Day	Breakfast	Lunch	Dinner	Snack
Day 29	Low-FODMAP Smoothie Bowl with Kiwi and Pineapple	Low-FODMAP Tofu Stir-Fry with Bok Choy	Roasted Turkey Breast with Low-FODMAP Gravy	Low-FODMAP Celery Sticks with Peanut Butter
Day 30	Oatmeal with Chia Seeds and Blueberries	Grilled Chicken Salad with Strawberries and Almonds	Low-FODMAP Shepherd's Pie with Sweet Potato Topping	Low-FODMAP Trail Mix with Almonds and Dark Chocolate

Days 31-40

Day	Breakfast	Lunch	Dinner	Snack
Day 31	Low-FODMAP Pumpkin Spice Muffins	Low-FODMAP Pasta Salad with Roasted Vegetables	Grilled Pork Chops with Quinoa and Green Beans	Rice Cakes with Peanut Butter and Banana Slices
Day 32	Poached Eggs on Gluten-Free Toast with Tomato Slices	Turkey and Swiss Lettuce Wraps	Low-FODMAP Eggplant Parmesan	Lactose-Free Yogurt with Blueberries
Day 33	Low-FODMAP Protein Pancakes with Maple Syrup	Low-FODMAP Thai Chicken Salad	Lemon Garlic Shrimp with Zucchini Noodles	Low-FODMAP Almond Butter Energy Balls
Day 34	Lactose-Free Cottage Cheese with Fresh Strawberries	Baked Tilapia with Lemon and Dill	Low-FODMAP Beef and Broccoli Stir-Fry	Low-FODMAP Apple Slices with Almond Butter

Day	Breakfast	Lunch	Dinner	Snack
Day 35	Baked Sweet Potato with Almond Butter and Cinnamon	Quinoa and Roasted Beet Salad	Baked Cod with Lemon and Roasted Asparagus	Carrot Sticks with Low-FODMAP Hummus
Day 36	Greek Yogurt with Low-FODMAP Fruit Compote	Low-FODMAP Chicken and Rice Soup	Low-FODMAP Chicken and Rice Casserole	Gluten-Free Pretzels with Low-FODMAP Guacamole
Day 37	Spinach and Cheddar Frittata	Grilled Vegetable and Hummus Sandwich	Grilled Lamb Chops with Quinoa Salad	Low-FODMAP Chia Pudding with Berries
Day 38	Rice Porridge with Cinnamon and Maple Syrup	Low-FODMAP Chicken and Avocado Salad	Low-FODMAP Stuffed Acorn Squash with Quinoa	Dark Chocolate Covered Strawberries
Day 39	Low-FODMAP Banana Nut Muffins	Rice Paper Rolls with Shrimp and Cucumber	Baked Chicken Breasts with Lemon and Rosemary	Low-FODMAP Trail Mix with Almonds and Dark Chocolate
Day 40	Scrambled Tofu with Bell Peppers and Spinach	Tuna Salad with Gluten-Free Crackers	Low-FODMAP Mushroom Risotto	Low-FODMAP Pumpkin Seed Granola Bars

Days 41-50

Day	Breakfast	Lunch	Dinner	Snack
Day 41	Low-FODMAP Blueberry Banana Pancakes	Grilled Chicken and Spinach Wraps	Grilled Lemon Herb Chicken with Quinoa	Lactose-Free Cheese and Grapes
Day 42	Spinach and Feta Omelette	Low-FODMAP Tomato and Basil Soup	Low-FODMAP Baked Salmon with Dill and Green Beans	Low-FODMAP Chia Pudding with Berries
Day 43	Low-FODMAP Overnight Oats with Strawberries	Rice Noodle Salad with Shrimp and Cucumber	Beef Stir-Fry with Bok Choy and Carrots	Rice Cakes with Peanut Butter and Banana Slices
Day 44	Quinoa Porridge with Maple and Pecans	Gluten-Free Turkey Club Sandwich	Low-FODMAP Chicken Alfredo with Gluten-Free Pasta	Low-FODMAP Almond Butter Energy Balls
Day 45	Low-FODMAP Avocado Toast on Gluten-Free Bread	Low-FODMAP Greek Salad with Feta and Olives	Stuffed Bell Peppers with Quinoa and Ground Beef	Low-FODMAP Trail Mix with Almonds and Dark Chocolate
Day 46	Scrambled Eggs with Spinach and Lactose-Free Cheese	Grilled Salmon with Quinoa and Asparagus	Low-FODMAP Shrimp and Vegetable Skewers	Carrot Sticks with Low-FODMAP Hummus

Day	Breakfast	Lunch	Dinner	Snack
Day 47	Rice Cakes with Peanut Butter and Banana Slices	Low-FODMAP Lentil Soup with Spinach	Baked Chicken Thighs with Sweet Potatoes	Gluten-Free Pretzels with Low-FODMAP Guacamole
Day 48	Coconut Yogurt Parfait with Low-FODMAP Granola	Baked Cod with Quinoa and Roasted Carrots	Low-FODMAP Vegetable Curry with Tofu	Low-FODMAP Celery Sticks with Peanut Butter
Day 49	Low-FODMAP Smoothie Bowl with Kiwi and Pineapple	Low-FODMAP Tofu Stir-Fry with Bok Choy	Roasted Turkey Breast with Low-FODMAP Gravy	Low-FODMAP Apple Slices with Almond Butter
Day 50	Oatmeal with Chia Seeds and Blueberries	Grilled Chicken Salad with Strawberries and Almonds	Low-FODMAP Shepherd's Pie with Sweet Potato Topping	Dark Chocolate Covered Strawberries

Days 51-60

Day	Breakfast	Lunch	Dinner	Snack
Day 51	Low-FODMAP Pumpkin Spice Muffins	Low-FODMAP Pasta Salad with Roasted Vegetables	Grilled Pork Chops with Quinoa and Green Beans	Lactose-Free Cheese and Grapes
Day 52	Poached Eggs on Gluten-Free Toast with Tomato Slices	Turkey and Swiss Lettuce Wraps	Low-FODMAP Eggplant Parmesan	Low-FODMAP Chia Pudding with Berries

Day	Breakfast	Lunch	Dinner	Snack
Day 53	Low-FODMAP Protein Pancakes with Maple Syrup	Low-FODMAP Thai Chicken Salad	Lemon Garlic Shrimp with Zucchini Noodles	Low-FODMAP Almond Butter Energy Balls
Day 54	Lactose-Free Cottage Cheese with Fresh Strawberries	Baked Tilapia with Lemon and Dill	Low-FODMAP Beef and Broccoli Stir-Fry	Low-FODMAP Apple Slices with Almond Butter
Day 55	Baked Sweet Potato with Almond Butter and Cinnamon	Quinoa and Roasted Beet Salad	Baked Cod with Lemon and Roasted Asparagus	Rice Cakes with Peanut Butter and Banana Slices
Day 56	Greek Yogurt with Low-FODMAP Fruit Compote	Low-FODMAP Chicken and Rice Soup	Low-FODMAP Chicken and Rice Casserole	Carrot Sticks with Low-FODMAP Hummus
Day 57	Spinach and Cheddar Frittata	Grilled Vegetable and Hummus Sandwich	Grilled Lamb Chops with Quinoa Salad	Low-FODMAP Trail Mix with Almonds and Dark Chocolate
Day 58	Rice Porridge with Cinnamon and Maple Syrup	Low-FODMAP Chicken and Avocado Salad	Low-FODMAP Stuffed Acorn Squash with Quinoa	Gluten-Free Pretzels with Low-FODMAP Guacamole

Day	Breakfast	Lunch	Dinner	Snack
Day 59	Low-FODMAP Banana Nut Muffins	Rice Paper Rolls with Shrimp and Cucumber	Baked Chicken Breasts with Lemon and Rosemary	Low-FODMAP Celery Sticks with Peanut Butter
Day 60	Scrambled Tofu with Bell Peppers and Spinach	Tuna Salad with Gluten-Free Crackers	Low-FODMAP Mushroom Risotto	Dark Chocolate Covered Strawberries

Long-term Health Management Advice

Maintaining a Balanced Diet Beyond LOW-FODMAP

When transitioning from the strict phase of the LOW-FODMAP diet, the goal is to reintroduce foods in a structured manner to maintain a balanced diet without triggering symptoms. This approach ensures you regain a wider variety of nutrients while identifying specific foods that exacerbate your condition.

The reintroduction phase is as critical as the elimination phase because it informs you about your body's tolerance to different FODMAPs. Start by reintroducing one food at a time, with a single serving, and monitor any changes in symptoms for three days. If there is no increase in symptoms, you can assume that food is safe for you and gradually increase its quantity or frequency in your diet. This process helps identify your personal threshold levels for various FODMAPs.

It's essential during this phase to maintain a well-organized food diary. This diary should not only track what you eat and the amounts but also any symptoms you experience. This detailed record-keeping can provide insights into which foods your body can handle and which ones you should continue to avoid or limit.

Diversifying your diet is crucial. The LOW-FODMAP diet can restrict the intake of certain fruits, vegetables, grains, and legumes, potentially leading to nutritional deficiencies if followed long-term without proper management. Aim to include a range of foods from all food categories after you have determined which foods are safe. Because of their diversity, you are certain to get a variety of nutrients, such as fiber, vitamins, and minerals that are vital to your general health.

Incorporating new foods slowly and methodically is also key to maintaining gut health. Introducing too many new foods at once can overwhelm your digestive system, making it difficult to pinpoint which food might be causing a problem if symptoms recur. Instead, add new foods one at a time and continue to monitor your body's response as you did during the reintroduction phase.

Working with a dietitian specialized in the LOW-FODMAP diet can be extremely beneficial during this phase. A dietitian can help tailor the reintroduction process to your specific needs, ensuring that you receive balanced nutrition and adequate intake of all essential nutrients. They can also assist in expanding your diet to include a broader array of foods while managing any digestive symptoms that arise.

Moreover, it's important not to let the process become a source of stress, as stress can itself exacerbate digestive symptoms. Finding ways to relax and manage anxiety, such as through meditation, yoga, or other stress-relief techniques, can be an integral part of managing your digestive health.

As you reintroduce foods, it's also beneficial to continue practices that support digestive health overall. These include regular exercise, which helps maintain normal gut function and reduces stress, and staying hydrated, which aids in digestion and prevents constipation.

Once you have successfully reintroduced various foods, it's critical to keep your diet as balanced and varied as possible. This not only ensures you get all the necessary nutrients but also helps maintain gut microbiota diversity, which is crucial for overall gut health. Eating a range of foods can help foster a resilient digestive system and reduce the likelihood of future gastrointestinal distress.

It's also valuable to stay updated on new research and recommendations in the field of gastroenterology and dietetics. Nutritional science evolves rapidly, and new discoveries about FODMAPs and digestive health can provide further insights that might adjust your approach to eating and managing symptoms.

Supplements and Nutrients: What You Need to Know

Following a restrictive diet like the LOW-FODMAP can sometimes result in nutritional gaps due to the elimination of various foods. It's crucial for individuals on this diet to be aware of potential deficiencies and consider incorporating certain supplements and nutrients to maintain their health.

The possibility of consuming less fiber when following the LOW-FODMAP diet is one of the main issues. Because it promotes healthy gut flora and helps control bowel motions, fiber is essential for digestive health. It might be difficult to get adequate fiber when there are limitations on some fruits, vegetables, and whole grains. A low-FODMAP fiber supplement that can help close this gap without aggravating symptoms is psyllium husk.

Calcium is another nutrient that might be in short supply on the LOW-FODMAP diet, especially if dairy products are limited or excluded due to lactose intolerance. Calcium is vital for bone health, nerve transmission, and muscle function. Calcium-fortified non-dairy alternatives like almond milk, lactose-free yogurt, or supplements can be good options to ensure adequate calcium intake.

Along with supporting bone health, vitamin D also helps with immunological response and reduces inflammation. It is strongly correlated with calcium. A vitamin D insufficiency may result from restricted sun exposure and food choices. Taking a supplement can help you maintain adequate amounts of vitamin D, which is especially important during the darker winter months.

Many individuals on restrictive diets might also find themselves low in B vitamins, particularly vitamin B12, which is commonly found in foods like meat, seafood, and dairy—products that might be limited on the LOW-FODMAP diet. B12 is necessary for healthy nerves as well as the synthesis of DNA and red blood cells. You may make sure you get a broad spectrum of B vitamins, including folate, which is crucial for those who are still fertile, by taking a B-complex vitamin supplement.

A further risk is iron deficiency, which is more common in women and those following a vegetarian or vegan LOW-FODMAP diet since red meat contains the most absorbable types of iron. Iron deficiency symptoms include weakness, exhaustion, and pale complexion. Iron supplements may be required if these symptoms are present, but they should be taken under a doctor's supervision as too much iron can be dangerous.

Magnesium is a mineral that is vital for muscle function, nerve function, blood glucose control, and blood pressure regulation. It's also important for the production of protein, bone, and DNA. Some people might find it hard to get enough magnesium from a LOW-FODMAP diet, as many magnesium-rich foods like legumes and certain nuts are high in FODMAPs. Supplementing with magnesium can help alleviate these gaps.

Zinc is crucial for immune function, wound healing, DNA synthesis, and cell division. It's another nutrient that can be limited on restrictive diets, especially vegetarian or vegan ones, as high-FODMAP foods like certain seeds and legumes are also good sources of zinc. Considering a zinc supplement might be beneficial if dietary intake is inadequate.

Good sources of omega-3 fatty acids, which are essential for reducing inflammation and preserving cardiovascular health, include walnuts, flaxseeds, and oily salmon. An omega-3 supplement made from fish oil or algae may be helpful if the diet excludes these foods.

Lastly, as dietary modifications may have an impact on the balance of gut flora, a probiotic supplement may be used to maintain it. Probiotics can improve general digestive health and the gut flora.

When considering supplements, it's important to choose high-quality products and discuss their use with a healthcare provider, especially since supplements can interact with medications and may not be necessary or suitable for everyone. Frequent blood tests can aid in detecting any nutritional deficits, guaranteeing that the diet is well-balanced and efficient in treating symptoms without endangering general health. This careful management ensures that while the diet controls digestive symptoms, it also supports robust overall health.

Building a Sustainable Healthy Lifestyle

Integrating the LOW-FODMAP diet into a sustainable lifestyle involves more than just managing what you eat. It's about creating a balanced approach that includes exercise, stress management, and good sleep practices, ensuring not only gastrointestinal health but overall well-being.

Starting with exercise, incorporating regular physical activity into your routine can significantly enhance digestive health. Exercise helps speed up digestion and can reduce symptoms of IBS, such as bloating and constipation. However, the key is to choose activities that you enjoy and can maintain regularly without feeling overwhelmed. Moderate activities like walking, cycling, swimming, or yoga can be particularly beneficial. Yoga, for instance, not only supports physical health but also aids in stress reduction and improves gastrointestinal function by enhancing gut motility.

Stress management is another crucial element when living with dietary restrictions. Prolonged stress can worsen symptoms of dyspepsia and increase the difficulty of adhering to a restricted diet. Stress-reduction methods, including progressive muscle relaxation, deep breathing exercises, and mindfulness meditation, can be quite effective. These techniques assist in lessening the physical symptoms of stress, such as IBS flare-ups, as well as the psychological effects of having a digestive disease.

Good sleep hygiene is also integral to sustaining a healthy lifestyle on the LOW-FODMAP diet. Insufficient sleep can impede the body's capacity to properly process and assimilate nutrients, resulting in heightened symptoms. Improved sleep quality may be attained by sticking to a regular sleep schedule, clearing out devices and other distractions from the bedroom, and maybe implementing nightly rituals like reading or having a warm bath. Avoiding stimulants like caffeine in the evening will help you have a more restful night and lessen sleep issues.

Diet-wise, while the LOW-FODMAP diet is restrictive in the initial phases, it is designed to be temporary. The goal is to reintroduce foods gradually and identify personal triggers. This can and should be done thoughtfully and systematically, adding one food at a time in small quantities and observing how your body reacts. Keeping a detailed food diary during this phase can help track which foods exacerbate symptoms and which are tolerated well.

It's also vital to ensure that the diet remains nutritionally balanced. Consulting with a registered dietitian who specializes in the LOW-FODMAP diet can provide you with tailored advice and meal plans that cover all nutritional bases. They can help ensure that while you manage your digestive symptoms, you're also getting a full range of nutrients essential for health.

Furthermore, as you adjust to integrating the LOW-FODMAP diet into your lifestyle, it can be helpful to prepare meals in advance. Meal prepping can help alleviate the stress of finding appropriate meals within the diet's restrictions, especially when you are busy or tired. It can also prevent situations where you might choose less healthy or symptom-triggering foods simply because they are more convenient.

Another aspect of sustainable living with the LOW-FODMAP diet is the social component. Dining out or eating at friends' homes can be challenging when following a strict dietary regimen. Educating friends and family about your dietary restrictions and planning ahead when eating out—such as reviewing menus in advance or contacting restaurants to discuss your dietary needs—can help maintain a social life and make the diet more manageable.

Lastly, stay informed about new research and resources on the LOW-FODMAP diet and IBS. The science surrounding digestive health is always evolving, and new findings can offer additional strategies to improve your health or make managing your diet easier.

By integrating these strategies into your routine, you can build a sustainable and healthy lifestyle that supports both your digestive and overall health. It's about making informed choices that fit your needs and enhance your quality of life in a holistic and balanced way.

Emotional Well-being Tips

Stress Management Techniques

Managing stress is crucial for individuals dealing with Irritable Bowel Syndrome (IBS), as stress can significantly exacerbate symptoms. Here are several practical stress management techniques that can help alleviate IBS symptoms and improve overall well-being:

1. **Mindfulness Meditation:** This technique involves sitting quietly and paying attention to thoughts, sounds, the sensations of breathing, or parts of the body. Mindfulness can help you become more aware of your stress and anxiety, allowing you to manage them more effectively. Regular mindfulness practice has been shown to reduce the impact of stress on the body and can specifically help in managing the anxiety that often accompanies IBS.

2. **Progressive Muscle Relaxation (PMR):** PMR involves gradually tensing and then relaxing different muscle groups in the body. This practice helps you become more aware of physical sensations and aids in relaxing the muscle tension that stress can cause. Since muscle tension is common in IBS, PMR can be particularly beneficial.

3. **Regular Exercise:** One of the best ways to alleviate stress is to exercise. It can lessen the worry and sadness that IBS frequently causes. Exercises that increase heart rate and reduce pain, such as

walking, cycling, swimming, or yoga, might cause the body to produce endorphins. IBS sufferers may benefit greatly from yoga's dual emphasis on gentle movements and breathing exercises.

4. **Deep Breathing Exercises:** Deep diaphragmatic breathing is an effective way to calm the nervous system and reduce the symptoms of stress. It involves focusing on slow, deep, and consistent breaths, which can help manage the immediate symptoms of stress.
5. **Cognitive Behavioral Therapy (CBT):** CBT is a helpful strategy for stress management because it can alter unfavorable cognitive patterns and behavior that exacerbate stress and symptoms of IBS. It can support the development of more effective coping strategies for anxiety and stress.
6. **Adequate Sleep:** IBS symptoms might worsen as a result of stress and inadequate sleep. Stress management may be greatly enhanced by establishing a pattern that encourages excellent sleep hygiene, such as minimizing screen time before bed, setting up a cozy sleeping environment, and maintaining regular wake and sleep periods.
7. **Guided Imagery:** This method of relaxing entails creating mental pictures to transport oneself to a tranquil, serene environment. Your body seems to react as though what you are picturing is true when you use all of your senses. Guided imagery can help someone with IBS picture their digestive system as peaceful and efficient.
8. **Diet Management:** Stress can also be managed by maintaining a stable blood sugar level. Avoiding large meals, reducing the intake of high-sugar foods, and increasing your water intake can prevent the stress associated with sudden spikes and drops in blood sugar levels.
9. **Journaling:** Expressing your ideas and feelings via writing might help you feel less stressed and better about yourself. This can be very useful for comprehending and controlling the feelings associated with having IBS.

10. **Connecting with Others**: It might help to lessen the loneliness that comes with having IBS to share your experiences and feelings with friends, family, or support groups. Just talking about your difficulties can sometimes bring relief and new strategies for handling stress.

You can better manage your stress and, consequently, lessen the symptoms of IBS and enhance your quality of life by implementing these techniques into your daily routine. It might be beneficial to experiment with several methods to see which ones work best for you, as every person's reaction to stress and IBS is different.

Mindful Eating: Connecting with Your Food

The practice of mindful eating entails giving your whole attention to the eating and drinking experience, both within and outside of your body. It teaches you to become conscious of the thoughts and feelings that surface throughout a meal, as well as the physical and subtle signals connected with eating, such as the textures, tastes, colors, and scents of food. Bringing non-judgmental awareness to your eating patterns, desires, bodily hunger, and satiety indicators is the goal of this mindfulness meditation technique.

The benefits of mindful eating are particularly significant for those dealing with digestive health issues like IBS. By eating mindfully, you can better regulate the way you eat, which can improve digestive symptoms. This happens because mindful eating slows down the eating process and can lead to better chewing and smaller bites, which aid digestion and absorption of nutrients. Chewing food thoroughly and slowly lessens the amount of work your digestive system has to perform to process it, which can help minimize indigestion and bloating sensations.

Furthermore, mindful eating helps you tune into your body's hunger signals and avoid overeating, which is often a trigger for digestive discomfort. By recognizing when you are actually hungry versus when you are eating out of boredom, stress, or sadness, you can begin to break the cycles of emotional eating that so often exacerbate digestive disorders.

Emotional regulation is another significant benefit of mindful eating. This practice can help you understand the emotional connections you have with food, which can be particularly powerful for people who suffer from gastrointestinal issues linked to stress and anxiety. By addressing these emotions directly, mindful eating can lessen the impact they have on your digestive health.

Overall, mindful eating encourages a harmonious relationship with food, which can be profoundly beneficial for long-term digestive health and general well-being. It allows individuals to enjoy their meals more fully and to use their body's cues to guide their eating habits in a healthier, more balanced way.

Low Fodmap grocery shopping list

Creating a detailed LOW-FODMAP grocery shopping list can help make meal planning and shopping easier for those managing digestive sensitivities.

Vegetables:

- Carrots
- Cucumbers
- Bell peppers (red and green)
- Zucchini
- Eggplant
- Potatoes
- Spinach
- Kale
- Green beans
- Tomatoes

- Ginger
- Olives
- Lettuce
- Chives
- Fennel (the bulb part)

Fruits:

- Unripe bananas
- Blueberries
- Strawberries
- Raspberries
- Oranges
- Kiwi
- Pineapple
- Grapes
- Cantaloupe
- Honeydew melon
- Lemon
- Lime

Proteins:

- Eggs
- Firm tofu
- Tempeh
- Chicken (fresh, not marinated)
- Beef (fresh cuts)

- Pork (fresh cuts)
- Fish (fresh or frozen without added seasonings)
- Shellfish (fresh)

Dairy and Alternatives:

- Lactose-free milk
- Lactose-free yogurt
- Hard cheeses (e.g., cheddar, Swiss)
- Almond milk (unsweetened)
- Coconut milk (for cooking, not canned)
- Rice milk (unsweetened)

Grains and Cereals:

- Gluten-free bread
- Rice (white, brown)
- Oats (gluten-free)
- Quinoa
- Corn (polenta, tortillas)
- Gluten-free pasta
- Sourdough spelt bread

Nuts and Seeds:

- Almonds (small serving)
- Walnuts
- Macadamia nuts
- Peanuts
- Pumpkin seeds

- Chia seeds
- Flaxseeds
- Sunflower seeds (small serving)

Condiments and Spices:

- Olive oil
- Coconut oil
- Garlic-infused oil
- Ginger-infused oil
- Vinegar (except apple cider vinegar)
- Mustard
- Mayonnaise (check for additives)
- Salt and pepper
- Most herbs (such as basil, cilantro, parsley)
- Spices (such as turmeric, cumin, coriander, paprika)

Snacks and Others:

- Gluten-free crackers
- Rice cakes
- Popcorn (plain)
- Dark chocolate (small quantities)
- Maple syrup
- Rice syrup

Beverages:

- Water (still or sparkling)
- Herbal teas (e.g., peppermint, ginger)

- Coffee (limit to small amounts)

This LOW-FODMAP shopping list provides a variety of food options that can help manage digestive symptoms while ensuring a balanced and nutritious diet. It is important to keep an eye out for high-FODMAP additions, such as powdered onions or garlic, and to watch portion sizes because even LOW-FODMAP meals can cause symptoms if ingested in excess.

Food to avoid and food to eat

The LOW-FODMAP diet is specifically formulated to alleviate symptoms associated with digestive disorders like irritable bowel syndrome (IBS). This diet minimizes the intake of foods high in certain carbohydrates known as FODMAPs, which can ferment in the gut and lead to discomforts such as bloating, gas, and abdominal pain.

High-FODMAP foods, including onions and garlic, are often recommended to avoid due to their high fructan content, which can ferment in the gut, causing discomfort. Wheat products like bread, pasta, and cereals that contain gluten and fructans should also be limited. Fruits such as apples, pears, cherries, and peaches are high in fructose, a simple sugar that some individuals struggle to absorb effectively, leading to symptoms. Additionally, vegetables like cauliflower, asparagus, and mushrooms contain polyols and fructans, which are also known to exacerbate symptoms. Legumes and pulses, including beans, lentils, and chickpeas, are rich in galacto-oligosaccharides, another category of FODMAPs that are difficult to digest for many. Dairy products containing lactose, such as milk, soft cheeses, and yogurt, can also trigger digestive issues in those with lactose intolerance.

Conversely, the diet encourages the consumption of low-FODMAP foods. Eggs and meats, being free from carbohydrates, do not contain FODMAPs and are excellent protein sources. Vegetables such as carrots, cucumbers, lettuce, and tomatoes are low in FODMAPs and generally well tolerated.

Fruits like oranges, grapes, and strawberries offer a sweet option without excessive fructose. Lactose-free dairy products and alternatives like almond milk or hard cheeses are suitable substitutes. Grains such as rice, quinoa, and gluten-free bread are also recommended as they are devoid of high-FODMAP components like fructans.

By adhering to these guidelines, individuals can better manage their dietary triggers and reduce symptoms, supporting not only symptom relief but also ensuring a nutritionally balanced diet. This approach empowers individuals to manage their condition effectively while enjoying a diverse and nutritious diet.

CONCLUSION

How to Stay Informed About New Research and Trends

Staying informed about the latest research and developments in digestive health and the LOW-FODMAP diet is essential for those managing digestive disorders and for health professionals providing guidance. The field of nutritional science is rapidly evolving, with new findings continually reshaping dietary recommendations and treatments.

To begin, regularly checking in with trusted medical websites that specialize in gastroenterology and nutrition can be invaluable. Websites such as those run by major hospitals, university research centers, or government health departments often provide updates on the latest research and guidelines in digestive health. These platforms frequently summarize recent studies, making it easier for non-specialists to understand the implications and practical applications of new discoveries.

Subscribing to medical journals like the "American Journal of Gastroenterology" or "Gut" is another effective way to access the most recent scientific research. Many journals offer lay summaries or newsletters that highlight key findings relevant to conditions like IBS and the effectiveness of diets such as LOW-FODMAP. For those who prefer a less technical approach, subscribing to newsletters from digestive health foundations and associations can provide updates in a more digestible format.

Engaging with online forums and social media groups focused on digestive health can also be beneficial. These communities often discuss the latest trends, share personal experiences, and provide support. Furthermore, attending webinars, workshops, and conferences on nutrition and digestive health can offer deeper insights and the opportunity to connect with experts in the field.

Lastly, consulting with healthcare providers during regular check-ups can help integrate the latest research findings into your management plan. Dietitians and gastroenterologists can offer personalized advice that reflects current best practices, ensuring that dietary strategies like the LOW-FODMAP diet are both effective and up-to-date.

By utilizing these resources, individuals can stay well-informed about advancements in digestive health, empowering them to make educated decisions about their diet and overall health strategy.

Staying abreast of the latest research and developments in digestive health and the LOW-FODMAP diet is crucial for anyone managing digestive disorders, as well as for healthcare professionals guiding patients through these conditions. The field of nutritional science and gastroenterology is dynamic, with continuous advancements that can significantly influence treatment protocols and dietary recommendations.

For individuals coping with digestive issues, understanding and integrating new research into daily management strategies can enhance the effectiveness of dietary interventions and improve quality of life. Below are several strategies to help keep informed about the latest in digestive health and the LOW-FODMAP diet:

Leverage Academic and Medical Journals

Academic and medical journals are primary sources for the latest research in digestive health. Journals such as the *American Journal of Gastroenterology*, *Gut*, and *Digestive Diseases and Sciences* regularly publish studies that explore various aspects of digestive health, including the efficacy of the LOW-FODMAP diet. Most journals offer abstracts that summarize study results, which are helpful for those without a background in medical science. For more in-depth information, full articles are available, although some may require a subscription or access through academic institutions or libraries.

Follow Reputable Health Websites and Blogs

Many reputable health websites and specialized gastroenterology blogs provide updates on recent research, often discussing how new findings can be practically applied. Websites such as Mayo Clinic, WebMD, or specific gastrointestinal disorder advocacy groups like the International Foundation for Gastrointestinal Disorders (IFFGD) offer resources and articles written to be accessible to the general public. These platforms often break down complex scientific data into key points that can be easily understood and applied by those affected.

Engage with Professional Networks

Joining professional networks or associations related to nutrition and gastroenterology can provide regular updates through conferences, seminars, and newsletters. Organizations like the Academy of Nutrition and Dietetics in the United States and similar bodies worldwide offer memberships to professionals and often to the public, providing resources that are vetted and reliable. Attending conferences, either in-person or virtually, can also provide insights into the latest research and practical applications directly from experts in the field.

Utilize Social Media and Forums

Social media platforms and online forums can be valuable for real-time information sharing and discussions. Many researchers and healthcare professionals share their findings directly through platforms like LinkedIn, Twitter, or ResearchGate. Additionally, forums dedicated to IBS and the LOW-FODMAP diet can offer community support and a chance to learn from others' experiences. It’s important, however, to verify the credibility of the sources and information shared in these less formal settings to avoid misinformation.

Subscribe to Newsletters

Many digestive health institutes, research centers, and health bloggers offer newsletters that summarize recent advancements and research in the field. It is simple to keep informed without actively seeking out new information by subscribing to these newsletters, which may provide a steady stream of current information straight to your inbox.

Regular Consultations with Healthcare Providers

Regular visits to your gastroenterologist, dietitian, or nutritionist provide opportunities to discuss the latest research findings and their implications for your treatment plan. Healthcare professionals typically have access to the latest studies and clinical guidelines, ensuring that the advice given is based on the most recent evidence.

Participate in Patient Advocacy Groups

Patient advocacy groups often have resources for education and support, and they may conduct their own research. These groups work to improve the lives of those affected by digestive disorders through advocacy, education, and research. Involvement with these groups can provide updates on new treatments, dietary strategies, and upcoming studies where you could potentially participate.

Educational Platforms and Online Courses

Enrolling in online courses or watching lectures about digestive health can also be an effective way to stay informed. Platforms like Coursera, Udemy, or even specific university websites offer courses in nutrition and health that include segments specifically about managing digestive health and understanding diets like LOW-FODMAP.

By using these techniques, people who are struggling with digestive illnesses, those who are caring for them, and medical professionals may all remain up to date on the most recent developments in digestive health research and trends. With this information, people may not only treat the illness more successfully but also take charge of their health and nutrition, taking a proactive approach to maintaining good digestive health.

Looking Forward: Your Path to a Healthier, Happier Life

Embracing the journey to better health, particularly when dealing with digestive issues, can often feel daunting and solitary. However, it's important to recognize that you are not alone in this journey. There is a vast community of individuals who share similar challenges, and an abundance of resources and support systems are designed to aid you in navigating this path. With each step, remember that you are moving towards a healthier, happier life, and each challenge faced is a stepping stone to understanding your body better.

Navigating a condition like IBS or other digestive disorders requires courage and patience. It's a personal journey that involves learning what works best for your body. This learning process is not just about identifying foods that you can enjoy without discomfort but also about understanding how your body responds to different stressors, including food, stress, and even excitement. Embracing this journey with optimism involves acknowledging that setbacks are part of the learning curve, not the end of the road.

The power of community in this journey cannot be overstated. Across the globe, countless others are facing similar struggles. Social media platforms, online forums, and support groups provide places where people may exchange stories, advice, and encouragement. These communities can be invaluable sources of emotional support and practical advice. They remind us that our struggles are shared and that collective wisdom can help lighten our individual burdens.

Furthermore, advancements in medical research and dietary management continue to evolve, bringing new insights and hope. Researchers are relentlessly working toward a better understanding of digestive health, and each new study provides further clarity and guidance. By taking advantage of these developments, you may improve your quality of life by making well-informed decisions.

Support is also available from healthcare providers who specialize in digestive health. Dietitians, gastroenterologists, and therapists can provide personalized care that respects your unique needs and lifestyle choices. These professionals not only offer medical advice and treatment but also provide reassurance and validation of your experiences. Their expertise can be a beacon of light on your path, illuminating the way forward and helping you navigate the complexities of dietary and lifestyle modifications.

As you move forward, take each day as a new opportunity to learn more about your body and what makes it thrive. Celebrate the small victories—perhaps a day free of discomfort or a successful introduction of a new food. These successes, however small they might seem, are milestones on your journey to recovery and health.

Embracing a proactive attitude towards life changes, including diet and stress management, plays a critical role in managing digestive health. Techniques such as mindful eating, regular physical activity, and stress reduction practices are not just strategies but also investments in your long-term health. They require consistent effort, but the rewards—improved health and increased happiness—are worth every step.

Remember, the goal is not just to manage symptoms but to thrive despite them. With the right tools and community support, you can navigate your health challenges with confidence and optimism. This journey, though fraught with challenges, is also filled with potential for renewal and growth. Each step forward, guided by knowledge and supported by a community, is a step towards a fuller, more vibrant life.

In closing, take heart in knowing that you have the strength and resources to improve your health and well-being. Your path may be difficult at times, but it is also paved with opportunities for success and moments of joy. Stay informed, stay connected, and, most importantly, stay hopeful. The road to a healthier, happier life is within reach, and with each small step, you are closer to achieving your wellness goals. Accept this trip with the knowledge that you are capable of handling anything that comes your way and that you will succeed with the help of your community.

Scan the QR Code and access your 3 bonuses in digital format

🔥 Bonus 1: 60 Day Meal Plan

🔥 Bonus 2: Emotional Well-being Tips

🔥 Bonus 3: Low Fodmap grocery shopping list

Made in United States
Troutdale, OR
11/15/2024

24849627R00066